AT HER FEET

AT HER FEET

POWERING YOUR FEMDOM RELATIONSHIP

by TammyJo Eckhart and Fox

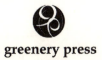

greenery press

© 2010 by Greenery Press, Inc.

All rights reserved. Except for brief passages quoted in newspaper, magazine, radio, television or Internet reviews, no part of this book may be reproduced in any form or by any means, electronic or mechanical, including photocopying or recording or by information storage or retrieval system, without permission in writing from the Publisher.

Cover design by Johnny Ink.

Published in the United States by Greenery Press, P.O. Box 5280, Eugene, OR 97405, www.greenerypress.com.

Distributed by SCB Distributors, Gardena, CA.

Readers should be aware that dominance and submission, like all sexual activities, carries an inherent risk of physical and/or emotional injury. While we believe that following the guidelines set forth in this book will minimize that potential, the writers and publisher encourage you to be aware that you are taking some risk when you decide to engage in these activities, and to accept personal responsibility for that risk. In acting on the information in this book, you agree to accept that information as is and with all faults. Neither the authors, the publisher, nor anyone else associated with the creation or sale of this book is responsible for any damage sustained.

CONTENTS

Introduction: Welcome to Life Like You Can't Imagine It, 1

1. TammyJo: Creation of a Femdom, 5
   Nature or Nurture? 5

2. Fox: Creation of a malesub, 11

3. How Two Became More, 17

4. Making M/s work every day, 27
   Basic Ideas Before You Start 27
   Getting Past the Search for "The One" 27
   Personal Expectations at the Beginning 29
   The Meaning of Consensual Slavery 33
   Slave Does Not Equal Submissive 36
   The Role of "Love" 42
   "Hurt" does not Equal "Harm" 47

5. Some Recommended Components, 55
   Contracts 55
   Rituals, Rules, & Protocols 58
   Training 65

6. Foundations of Owner/slave Dynamics, 73
   Commitment 73
   Loyalty 75
   Selfishness 77
   Obedience 82
   Needs & Wants 85
   Fetishes: A Special Type of Want 88
   Privacy 95
   Play Time 99

7   Daily Realities: Adjusting & Maintaining the Dynamic, 103
      Economic Realities *103*
      Social Expectations *108*
      Poly or Mono Structure *115*
      Sex *121*
      Illness & Injuries *126*
      Emotional and Mental Health *130*
      Family & Friends *135*
      Examples of Everyday D/s and Ownership *140*

8   Paradoxes of Owner-slave Dynamics, 145
      Using and Needing Your Slave: The Paradox of Ownership *143*
      Active Submission: the Paradox of Slavery *145*

TammyJo's Concise Advice for Femdoms, 147

Fox's Concise Advice for malesubs, 149

Appendix: Sample Contracts, 151

INTRODUCTION

WELCOME TO LIFE LIKE YOU CAN'T IMAGINE IT

Have you ever asked yourself these questions about femdom relationships?

- *Is love necessary?*
- *How important is sex?*
- *Do I have to have rules, protocols and rituals?*
- *How true are these porn images I see?*
- *Will my fetish get in the way of my relationship?*
- *Are slaves powerless?*
- *Are mistresses always right?*
- *How many of my family and friends will I lose if I do this 24/7?*
- *How can I be in the mood if I'm worried about money?*
- *Does the D/s have to stop if I'm sick?*
- *How can I become a better slave or mistress?*

These are just some of the questions we will address in *At Her Feet: Powering Your Femdom Relationship*. We will tackle all the traditional questions about setting up your dominant and submissive or mistress and slave relationship, but also look honestly at how all this kinky stuff works day in and day out for years. For us, the authors, we've made just this one mistress-slave relationship work for over a decade, and that is only the most recent relationship we've successfully had.

We think you've picked up this book because you're looking for a femdom relationship. Perhaps you're a submissive man who wants to know he isn't alone in his desires and wonders why he can't meet that kinky lady of his dreams. You may be a dominant woman who feels frustrated by the choices you seem to be offered in the BDSM community or the mass media, and you too are wondering where that kneeling knight is in your life.

You may also be picking up this book because you are in such a relationship, but you're concerned it isn't going to last beyond the first few passionate months. Perhaps you've been together for a year or two and you feel like things are going stale.

We've been there, right where you are. We understand your feelings and thoughts. We also understand the desire to just find that perfect someone and settle down.

Between the two of us we have more than 30 years of experience in BDSM, over ten years of that in a committed M/s or 24/7 femdom relationship. We want to share with you how we got to this place and the truths we've learned about ourselves, our community, and the society that raised us. While no one else will have an identical journey, we believe our experiences, work, and reflections may offer you insights into becoming the best mistress and the best slave you can become. Along the way we're going to challenge several of the most common ideas about BDSM, because sometimes belief in these concepts is a hurdle to creating an M/s dynamic and can damage your ability to maintain M/s for a continuous period.

A femdom and malesub relationship that goes beyond sex, beyond playtime, and into the everyday for years and years requires courage from both parties. If you have that courage or want to learn how to find it in yourself, keep reading. By the time you are finished with this book, you will have a better idea of how to power your own relationship and make it work for you and yours.

First, let us briefly introduce ourselves and what you will find in these pages.

TammyJo Eckhart, PhD, is an ancient historian by training, a teacher by personality, a dominant by nature, and a published fiction author by fate. She has over 20 years of committed experience in BDSM. The chapter "The Creation of a Femdom" isn't so much an autobiography as a reflection on the common experiences of many female dominants she's met, experiences that led them to their identity as dominants in BDSM relationships with a desire to go beyond the bedroom and into a life of D/s.

Fox graduated with a BS degree in physics with minors in both mathematics and psychology. He began investigating BDSM as a young adult in an effort to understand certain personal drives and fantasies that seemed to differ from those of his peers. His exploration led him through enough useful information and baseless crap to tell the difference fairly readily. In the chapter "The Creation of a Malesub," he'll share some of the story behind how he and others of his generation recognized their kinkiness and found avenues to pursue it.

TammyJo and Fox have been together in some form of D/s or M/s relationship since the autumn of 1999. We talk more about how we met and what led us into our mistress-slave life in chapter 3, "How Two Became More." This is part autobiography, but primarily we want to share the challenges and rewards of our early relationship that may mirror your own, or at least provide an honest image of how these relationships can begin.

The bulk of this book, Chapter 4, is "Making Femdom Work Every Day," focusing on how we make this work, day in and day out, year after year, through some serious challenges. The truths we've learned, sometimes with a great deal of struggle, will highlight what we know are common issues for all M/s and 24/7 dynamics as well as point out the unique challenges that can face femdoms and malesubs living in a western society. Just like life, we will cover the lovely kinky things and the necessary, mundane matters that we face together. We will hold off on the purely titillating material but otherwise hold little back so you can learn from our mistakes and successes.

We do not talk about subjects such as illegal slavery, blackmail, the idea that slaves can't leave their owners, or the superiority of one sex/gender over another as the reason why one is a slave or an owner. This is a book about consensual adult relationships, even if an outsider may have difficulty seeing the consent. We'll say it again: This is about consensual adult relationships only. We will also not address topics with which we do not have personal experience, because we want to offer you the best advice so you can empower yourself and your dynamic. The best advice must come from two places: knowledge and experience. If we haven't studied it or reflected on it as well as experienced it, we won't be talking about it. Sometimes our stories and insights may seem far from your own, but we believe the truths we've uncovered can help anyone who wants to build their life on a foundation of D/s and power it through the years to come.

In this book we will try to use terms consistently, but the terms and abbreviations have changed over the years. What TammyJo learned as SM has turned into BDSM in many circles and has been further divided into SM, D/s, and BD, as well as a ton of other categories and classifications.

We will only use our former partners' first names with their permission. Otherwise you will see people identified only by scene names and initials. We will try to keep everything and everyone clear, but with over three decades of experience between us, things are complex. Authors, educators, and activists we've met, seen or read will be mentioned by their full names, and we hope they consider this our ode to them (plus some publicity to boot).

Remember when we mentioned this book is going to challenge some of the common ideas in BDSM? Let's start right now. You've likely heard that D/s (dominant-submissive) and M/s (master-slave) relationships are built on "power exchange," right?

Wrong! Go back and take a look at the title of this book. This entire book is designed to reveal the truth about that expression and show why it fails to help you create a happy full-time femdom relationship. We are going to look at how we each became empowered as individuals and how our mistress-slave dynamic continues to empower us as unique people, as a couple, as part of a polyamorous family, and as members of the BDSM community at large.

Why? Power is what gives you the ability to do anything. Without it, you can achieve nothing, so you can't lose it if you want to make a relationship work. To make your relationship thrive you must exercise, direct and enhance your power. What is often seen as the slave giving the mistress power is actually the recognition of her authority to direct that power — the slave must be the one to exercise the power itself, since there is very little she could do to force him to act. Slaves forced into action are unlikely to do their best or be their quickest because their hearts and minds are not in it. Every owner we've met wants the best and most efficient service possible, so needing to force the slave every day and night undermines the owner's goal (and leads to burnout).

Neither of us has lost or lent out our individual power. By working together toward the mutual goal of a healthy and successful M/s relationship, we help each other improve as people and as a couple, enhancing and increasing our power and therefore directing a higher quality and greater quantity of power toward the dynamic itself. Beyond just the two of us, this power expansion also gives us the foundation from which to contribute to the well-being of everyone around us.

This may sound like a radical idea, particularly when it's commonplace to call BDSM a "power exchange." Well, it is radical, and because this is such a radical idea, we will be returning to it over and over in this book.

To paraphrase something TammyJo has said for years: mistress-slave relationships are both more mundane than you can imagine, more intense than you may be able to handle, and more rewarding than you can grasp when you first begin. They are not for everyone.

If you think, if you hope, that a 24/7 femdom relationship where the woman consensually owns the other is right for you, keep reading and working your heart and head through these chapters.

1

TAMMYJO: CREATION OF A FEMDOM

NATURE OR NURTURE?

TammyJo writes: When it comes to female dominants, or femdoms if you like that catchphrase, I strongly believe our sexuality is a bit of both. Frankly, I believe there is probably a bit more nature at play, given that the vast majority of us grew up in patriarchal households and societies and still managed to not buy into the notion that being female was an illness or a liability, let alone that it made us subservient to others who just happen to have a penis. To believe that you should be the one in charge of your relationship without being a nagging shrew, or that you could even have a relationship where you didn't need to follow traditional gender roles, means that you had the strength of character and the willpower to look beyond the vast majority of the models of womanhood you were bombarded with day in and day out.

I want to highlight some of the events that may have signaled to you as they did to me that I wasn't the average woman just looking for a man to support her while she took care of him. I think you'll find some similarities to my life journey in your own as I look at the femdom child, the femdom teen, the femdom young adult and the mature femdom stages of my life.

As a child my mother always said that I was bossy. She was right. Even though we lived in a neighborhood where for many years I was the only girl, the boys followed my lead in the games we played and the roles we took. On those rare moments when a boy was the "leader," I found ways of subverting his authority within the confines of the scenario. For example, while a boy might be captain of our imaginary spaceship,

I was ship's doctor and didn't hesitate to declare him ill and confine him to sickbay if I disagreed with his decisions. When I played "Peter Pan," my Wendy didn't wait around to be rescued, which annoyed "Peter" to no end, and yet he still asked me to come over to his house to play the next day. When I took on leadership roles such as playing a teacher, I relished the power I had, but I also spent a good deal of time with my students, so they wanted to play over and over again.

The femdom as a girl will be strong-willed but also clever, because she can sense if not explicitly see that her ideas and behaviors may not match the roles her parents or community expect her to have. A naturally dominant child will attract playmates who want to be around her, and will not have to rely on bullying or material possessions to gain companions. In many aspects such a child will be patient and seem quite polite until someone attempts to do something she does not approve of, then she will state her case or simply walk away, pulling some of the play group with her.

The femdom child may also question gender roles as well as push the envelope of what is acceptable. I wore ties to school one year and rejected traditional feminine roles such as cheerleader to be on the quiz bowl team or student director of drama performances. Some femdom children will become official leaders, but often they are dissuaded from or simply denied those roles, so you'll find them in supportive roles such as class secretary or working with all-girl groups. Watching interactions where her wishes become the group's reveals the truth of who has the most influence.

Much of the femdom child's world, though, is conducted inside her head. In her imagination she may be the pirate captain or the president. This tendency showed up repeatedly in my creative writing as well as the topics I looked at in school for projects and papers. I couldn't see myself in the traditional feminine role models, so I went looking for tales of strong women. That these women were often punished by society for being strong made me angry, but didn't dissuade me from wanting to be like them. It also showed up in my play, where my female dolls bossed their male companions around and sometimes their female sidekicks, too. I automatically filtered pop culture like TV and books so that years later I couldn't remember episodes unless some man or boy was tied up or a girl or woman came to the rescue. Amazons were particularly likely to stand out in my memory, because they came from a society where women were in charge and that was considered normal.

The point here is that I was naturally dominant and assertive, but I had to find acceptable ways of expressing it as a child, because as a girl in the 1970s

I was not encouraged to be dominant. Independent, yes. Dominant, no. Just looking casually at me and my family you may not have seen it, but if you watched for a while, if you read what I wrote and talked to me, you would have seen the evidence of a strong dominant personality trapped by a more traditional family and community.

Several of these personality trends continued when I became a teenager, though society and biology also attempted to conspire against me. The teen years are a time of rapid, confusing change, but when you are naturally dominant and female they are even more so. The images of teen girls around me said I should dress "feminine" and that boys didn't like smart girls. Luckily I never gave in to the idea that I had to act dumb, but I wore some clothes that make me shudder today. I also seemed to defer to my boyfriends, but that was the image I presented in public and not a reflection of what was happening in private, where I made it clear what was and was not going to happen. I even went so far as to use severe sexual teasing and "feminine wiles" to get my way. I recall multiple times when I withheld intercourse with a vague idea that it might happen later if my boyfriend let me restrain his hands or got me something I wanted. Does that sound familiar to you ladies?

That's a tough tightrope to balance on, because you can use those "feminine wiles," but you can also get a reputation you may not want. You can continue to be smart and excel at school, but you may not get the quarterback to ask you out. Of course, the naturally dominant teen girl may not want the quarterback, instead being happy with the boys who are hoping to do things for her. Oh, I did indeed have boys who wanted to do things for me with never an attempt to ask me out or even try to get a kiss. They were like my first harem by the time I was a senior, a small clique of boys who literally followed me around. I took advantage of them, I really did, and I'm betting if you think back to your teenage years, you can see boys who were eager to follow you who you used as well.

I came to that realization as an adult several years ago, and it upset me. But as I thought more about it and learned more about psychology, sociology, and feminist analysis of society, I understood. Without the concepts of safe, sane and consensual readily available to me — and indeed these have only very recently and very rarely been discussed in a vanilla context — I had no way to know a better way of doing things. I graduated from high school in 1988, before personal computers were common, so my resources for finding information were limited. Those of you who are older than me may have had still fewer resources, while younger ladies will have had access to more information.

When I went to college at the beginning of my young adulthood, all of that changed. Suddenly I was in a location where the library had information about what I was doing, though it was mostly psychological studies that more often than not called it sick. I was also in classes where the ideas of gender and gender roles were discussed, and I felt I could talk about wanting to be in charge and, indeed, feeling like it was natural for me to be. I started trying to find all the information I could, but still found myself struggling between feminine role models and my own inclinations.

Some of you ladies reading may have put your dominant tendencies to the side at this stage of your life. Perhaps you simply couldn't find young men willing to let you direct things, or perhaps you decided your desires were "unnatural" and retreated to the traditional roles. Perhaps you just got so busy with family and career that surviving day to day took over your priorities. Maybe you never had opportunities to try out your ideas because of your family and community, so your desires remained buried deep inside. Nature isn't enough; you have to have a way to be nurtured as well.

In college, I was lucky in that I liked geeks a lot; in fact, I think of myself as one these days. I started dating the man I am now married to, Tom, and he knew a lot about computers and was getting on this new thing called the Internet. This was before the picture and video laden net we have today, when information was really just words. He found us the online communities where we could ask questions and realize we were not alone in our desires. Perhaps you've had this feeling too, before you found others online who liked to watch male characters get tied up on TV shows or who felt the Amazons may have had the correct social model for society. Online in the early 1990s, I wasn't surrounded by porn images of dominant women, but today it is quite different. Today you can barely find an online community where the sidebars aren't riddled with slave girls or so-called femdoms in collars and impossibly high heels screaming profanities at the rather ugly men cowering before them. I'm so glad that I didn't have those images in front of me when I was a young woman. I suspect, though, that a natural femdom online today must push through the porn like I pushed through patriarchy to make a place for myself.

Further complicationg all those challenges to becoming a female dominant is the fact that the young woman is still learning a lot about herself in every aspect of her life, from figuring out a career to balancing family and friends to dating to determining how much of what she was raised to believe is what she honestly believes. Where you live has a huge impact on what is available to help you learn to become a confident femdom. I was in a small city in the middle of the Midwest; I had to actively seek out information, and as I did, I learned to negotiate with my boyfriends instead of manipulating them.

I found my husband through our shared academic and arts interests, and we were married before I was anywhere near being a femdom. Many young women enter an established relationship before they fully embrace their natures as dominants. A supportive man can help you explore safely and may even encourage you to do so, as mine did. But my biggest growth as a femdom came when we moved to New York City, where I went to graduate school for five years.

Big cities often have BDSM organizations if you know how and where to look. But you can't just look; you have to get involved, and I did, joining two groups and helping to establish a university one called Conversio Virium[1]. I went to public dungeons and play parties, and I talked to anyone I felt had a skill or an idea I wanted to explore. Once you get that taste, you want more. You learn that knowledge is sexy and, of course, you want to be as sexy as possible to attract good-looking and nice submissive partners. You buy some, or perhaps a lot, of the "fetish" clothes, and you learn to love it or use it to help you set the stage for your scenes.

At this stage, which I'd call my first five years of consciously trying to find information and get involved in BDSM, the young femdom is utilizing a lot of the porn images of women. Why? Well, let's be honest; when you're younger you tend to have a better body that looks more like the images you see. But also you lack experience, so the clothes and the words you may use are an attempt to try out the models you see around you. You are in effect practicing at being a femdom at this stage. It is fun; you feel alive, and you are likely getting your heart broken a few times along the way.

In my experience, if you put yourself out there and get involved in your community, you start to figure out what really works for you and what doesn't, and then you can begin to make conscious decisions about what to reject from the femdom model and what to embrace. When you start simply being dominant, for example while wearing teddy bear slippers or torn sweatpants, and are still able to get your submissive to kneel at your feet with a mere word or look, you have crossed over to the mature stage of femdom development. In many ways this is a full-circle journey, getting back to what feels natural for you but with an awareness you didn't have when you were younger. You know that the words you use are most valuable when you know what makes that specific man tick. You

---

1 http://www.conversiovirium.org

know that the tone of your voice is more important than the volume. You know that feeling sexy is more important than the size of your bra or the length of your skirt. You certainly learn that your desires had better be your principal reason for doing any of this or you will burn out fast.

At this stage you may feel ready to settle down with one (or perhaps more) submissives; you might even start entertaining the idea of 24/7 or an owner-slave dynamic in your life. That is the stage of femdom development where this book will do you the most good. When you are ready to find and create a long-term relationship with someone else, founded on the ideas of your being in charge and his being of service, then this is the book for you. You may be relatively young, in your early twenties, or an older woman who recently discovered there are ways to express her dominant nature without being a bitch. Either works, because while these stages I discussed may feel familiar to many of us, the ages we went through them will vary greatly.

This has been a very shortened view of my own growth as a femdom, but now I want to introduce you to the journey of my slave, Fox, for all the submissive and bottom men out there.

2

FOX: CREATION OF A MALESUB

Fox writes: Before I begin, I should probably mention that when Mistress mentioned the concept for this book to me, I thought it was a great idea. When she mentioned how the few books talking about femdom relationships are written only from the dominant's perspective and how she thought it was important to include the perspective of the submissive as well, I agreed that it made perfect sense. When I realized that I was going to be the one to offer that perspective, however, I panicked.

Over the years, from my initial explorations, to my time doing education panels and workshops, to the many conventions I've attended with Mistress, I've met all sorts of different personalities who identified with my side of the D/s coin. With each broadening of my horizons, and the introspection that invariably followed, it's been tricky to avoid the occasional crisis of identity. I've met "pets" and "bottoms" with whom I seemed to share more in common than some "slaves." I've heard some describe their "slave soul" with almost religious intensity, while I had a hard enough time overcoming my personal stigma of associating myself with that title.

With my unique experiences, beliefs, and personality, I worried how anything I could say would be relevant to someone else in this type of relationship. I finally consoled myself that this would be true of any malesub participating in this project. So, there it is; I make no claim to being a representative of malesubs, no expert in male submission. My sole credential is that I've been in a rewarding D/s relationship for more than a decade now.

But how did I become a male submissive? I suppose it's more accurate to ask how I came to realize that's what I was. Unlike TammyJo, who was the youngest of several brothers and sisters, I was born into a small family as the younger brother of one sister. As I suspect is the case growing up in most close families, I was heavily influenced by the behaviors and personality traits of my parents and sibling.

My father, for example, was a strong and honorable man serving in the military. His work, sadly, kept him absent overseas for the better part of every year, but he did his best to maintain a presence with the family despite the distance. Besides his sense of humor, the traits he possessed that I see most in myself were his sense of honor and obligation. Growing up, I often heard adults make promises as though it was an alternative to saying "I'll try." If my father made a promise, however, he took it very seriously. I watched him on many occasions do everything in his power to fulfill his word and I can recall him failing only once despite his best efforts. Because he treated his promises so seriously, he rarely made them, and only made them if it was something he had control over and if he had every intention of following through. As a child, I witnessed the respect others showed my father for this trait and it left a big impression on me. So, like my father, I rarely make promises but when I promise Mistress something, she does not question it and visibly relaxes, knowing that the task will be done. This enables me to do the task without a string of interruptions and reminders and allows Mistress to move onto other things with peace of mind.

As for my mother, she had the determination one would expect from a woman juggling a job and the pressures of raising two children alone for the better part of every year. With so many things to do and remember as part of running a household, my mother was a skilled multi-tasker and a prolific list-maker. The quality that rubbed off on me, though, was organization. I learned that it was easier to do more – and do it better – if my surroundings were ordered. I also learned early on that the organization of space was linked to organization of time. For example, less time spent looking for shoes and jackets meant more time at the park. As an adult, those skills have allowed me to balance a job, a business, my relationship with Mistress as well as my duties as her assistant, my regular commitments, and still have free time for myself (very important for preventing burnout).

Finally, while definitely not the source, my sister quite likely contributed to my love of bondage play. According to my parents, from the day of my arrival in the family my sister viewed me as one of her toys. An extremely creative free spirit, my sister was adept at composing any number of captor/captive role-play scenarios where I was invariably the captive. The two I recall in greatest detail were being tied securely to a chair as the captured "secret agent" and one where I was sent to the "stockade" – which involved being shut up in my bedroom closet as she leaned against the door from the outside.

Now, of course my sister didn't do this to make me kinky. Like I said, she was not the source. In all honesty, I don't think I'll ever know what the awakening of my original love of being bound was. One of my earliest memories involved wrapping myself tightly in my bed sheets and comforter and feeling a tremendous sense of peace and safety. There was nothing sexual about it then, just a positive emotion, but it would change as I grew older, morphing and merging itself into my first sexual fantasies.

Like TammyJo, I saw some things on television and read some in books that resonated with me. The Universal Studios 1933 version of *The Mummy*, with the incomparable Boris Karloff, was one of these. In it, the character he plays is arrested for attempting to bring his love back from the dead using forbidden magic. For this, he is sentenced to be mummified and buried alive. What ensues is one and a half minutes of the most terrifying and exciting struggles ever captured on celluloid. I bought this movie when it was re-released on VHS as part of the studio's Halloween classics campaign. I bought several others as subterfuge, but The Mummy received the most watches by far. I honestly did enjoy the film in its entirety, but I often kept it cued to the beginning of that scene. I suppose what struck me about it was the disproportionate punishment for a guy who was acting out of immense grief. He's a little less of a sympathetic character after being revived (he's a monster, after all), but I imagine being buried alive in a nameless grave would cause anyone to become a little unhinged.

One of my more positive role models was MacGyver, mullet-sporting titular character of the 1980s television series. Beyond the fact he was always getting captured or finding himself in dangerous situations, I loved that he used his intellect and ingenuity to pull off most of his escapes, rather than brute force or lethal weapons. He also genuinely liked helping people out, never asking for an award for putting himself in harm's way. If I had to say where the core of my submission comes from, I'd have to say that's it. I'm not defusing bombs with neon signs and skim milk, but it feels good to be able to help other people, or a special person in particular, for no other reason than you have the willingness and ability to.

There were, however, several ways in which I didn't compare to my role model – or my parents' expectation of traditional gender roles. While my buddy "Angus" was physically tough and adept, emotionally hardened, and athletic,

I was physically scrawny, emotionally sensitive, and wholly disinterested in competing in sports. Sadly, I was the cerebral type (i.e., a huge nerd) and didn't grow up living around many children my own age, and the combination led to a number of socially awkward school years. I had a few friends and I got along well with peers with similar drives, like those in drama club, speech team, and academic bowl, but I definitely had a hard time following, participating in, or even caring about the animal kingdom-like rituals of high school courtship.

That changed quite unexpectedly in the summer before my 17th birthday. I was attending a summer science camp at the state university along with 20 other specially-selected students from high schools across the state. About the second night in, I was approached by a very pretty girl who happened to share a number of interests and opinions similar to my own. We hit it off very quickly and over the course of the next few months we were darn near inseparable. It was all very dizzying, especially for me as the experience was so novel. One thing I noticed as time went on was that my partner was the boss of the relationship. Her ideas tended to become our ideas. A lot of her ideas were good ones; others I wasn't very keen on, but I went ahead anyway because I wanted to keep her happy. I could have said no to this or that, but any resistance I may have had was displaced by my desire to keep her happy. When the summer was over, the relationship was over. It ended with me being told that it had all been fun, but that I had merely been a convenience. All I will say is that it hurt and it took a while to get over it.

When school started up again, life had another experience waiting for me. To my surprise, I was being pursued by another girl who was a year ahead of me. She had asked me out a few times, but I'd always had other commitments. Still feeling a little burned, I wasn't eager to enter into another relationship, but on the other hand, she did seem nice and several of my friends had begun urging me to take her to the junior prom. Long story short, I did take her to the prom and we had a fine time, but something that really stood out about her is that you couldn't get her to share her opinion on anything. She was deferent to the point of frustration. No matter how you phrased the question, her reply was always along the lines of "me too!" or "I don't know, which do you like?" or "whatever you want will be fine." The only winning move in this game was to be considerate, watch her body language, and assume she was happy unless indicated otherwise. It was exhausting.

Having experienced relationships with partners of such polarized differences in attitude and personality gave me a lot to consider. In spite of the increasing frequency and complexity of my erotic fantasies, I was fortunate to both realize – and be concerned by – just how easy it might be to get entangled in a harmful relationship. I knew the only way to avoid that was to learn everything I could about BDSM and define exactly what it was I was personally searching for (so that I could recognize it when I found it). Unfortunately, I knew from previous attempts that this was a lot more difficult than it sounded.

In the beginning, I had scoured our county library for books on sexuality and alternative lifestyles, but unsurprisingly, there was little to be found in such a conservative area about such taboo subjects. Most non-fiction literature that I was able to find addressed it in the context of abnormal psychology. Helpful books such as Miller and Devon's *Screw the Roses, Send Me the Thorns* and Jay Wiseman's *SM 101* were still fairly new and were certainly not in my local library. This left few good alternatives. While I had been surreptitiously exploring BDSM via the Internet since getting on-line, I knew enough to be skeptical; that is, the most prevalent and most easily-located sources were probably also the least reliable. Eventually, like TammyJo, I came across the USENET (similar to online Bulletin Board Systems and the precursor to modern web forums), but I found the way USENET operated to be both slow and frustrating.

From here I moved on to observing chatrooms via IRC (Internet Relay Chat). Most of what I saw was in the vein of roleplaying, with interactions modeled on the fictional settings of, and emphasizing the same details found in, a lot of Internet pornography. Some of it, however, was actually helpful. Several chat rooms actually had regulars who were couples offline and used IRC to stay in touch with other friends and couples they would usually only see at street fairs and conventions. I identified myself as a novice who was seeking to learn what they could teach me about BDSM, how others had discovered the community, and how different people practiced it in real life. I'm ashamed to say that I misrepresented myself as a freshman attending a college in the Midwest (since I was still many months away from eighteen), but I rationalized it to myself because it would eventually be true. While obviously I couldn't verify the veracity of their biographies either, the fact that there were nearly two dozen people with different IP addresses, whose statements corroborated with each other, caused me to lend a little more weight to their testimony.

Over the course of months, I found myself a welcome visitor to the channel. Most conversation was about everyday news and activities, but when BDSM-related subjects came up, the regulars were open to my questions and extremely patient when explaining whatever I didn't understand. In the end, however, it was clear that continuing my quest would require actually meeting and interacting in person with the people in the community.

My chance first came during the summer of my 18th birthday. Thanks to events earlier in the year, I was hired for a brief internship in Boston, Massachusetts. While not alone, I was about 800 miles from home and family, and that gave me the freedom to explore the area in my free time. About two weeks in, I found an alternative weekly tabloid left behind on an outdoor café table. Despite only having a half-hour left for my lunch break, I sat down immediately to skim through it. In the back was an advertisement for a rope-bondage demo scheduled to take place the next night at a local club that was so nearby I wondered how I'd missed it!

A little overeager considering I still didn't know how I was going to get in, I arrived to find the venue hadn't opened yet. Fortunately, a small group was already waiting and I struck up a conversation with them to pass the time. This turned out to be lucky for me because I managed to walk right in beside them when the club opened. That night, I saw exactly what I'd been waiting and hoping to see. The demonstration was made up of a male dominant and his female slave. While there was the expected D/s etiquette between them, there was obvious respect and open affection as well. As he began weaving her swimsuit-clad body into a beautiful harness of jute, they occasionally shared jokes and laughter with their audience (which I was observing just as intently). Toward the end, I even participated as he showed me how to perform a few of the simpler ties. It was so much fun! It was exhilarating!

It was comforting.

Despite the reassurance of my IRC mentors, up until that night I still had the nagging worry that there was nowhere I would fit in within the BDSM community, that I wasn't suited for it, and that there was no way that I could have my desires met without fundamentally altering my personality. This experience proved to me that a partnership could exist – one where both parties contributed and benefitted equally and both were respected by themselves and others in their roles as dominant and submissive. Most importantly, rather than having to be as serious as a heart attack all the time, it was possible to have a sense of humor.

Finally, I could define what I was searching for and knew how to recognize it. And now I also knew that once I was ready and able to look for it, it was out there.

3

HOW TWO BECAME MORE

We're sure you've heard the expression "the two become one" in regards to marriage. When TammyJo got married, she and Tom rejected the notion that one of them was disappearing or that they'd cease to be two wonderful individuals, and they wrote their own vow to reflect those beliefs. She continues to reject that notion of one person being subsumed into another in regards to D/s and M/s dynamics as well, even though as the dominant she'd be in the position of gaining the most. Or so it would seem. We'll talk more about this idea in the fourth chapter, but for right now it is important that you know she never wants her submissives or even slaves to cease to be the amazing people who attracted her notice, and thus when she accepts authority from them, "the two become more."

We're going to start this chapter with each of us recounting briefly how we met and what made us decide to start the process of training that led to this 11-year owner-slave relationship. Then we're going to write together about what that training involved, how our relationship developed, and how we even got to be in a 24/7 dynamic that has further changed into what it is today. We'll continue with "ladies first" to lessen any confusion to the reader.

TammyJo remembers: Two years after moving to Bloomington, I met Fox. It was the start of the second year of Headspace, another university group I was part of, and I was working as part of its steering committee and felt things were going well. We had a growing membership, the vice-president and I had recently been to a Leather Leadership Conference[1], and

---

1   http://www.leatherleadership.org

we had recently increased from one to two munches a month, along with a monthly workshop or lecture. That was great, because I was taking German in the evenings as the final language I needed for my PhD. This meant I was missing one of the monthly munches and always came in late to the workshop or lecture, but since I could make it to the other munch and others were running the events, I could do what I needed to do to succeed academically while still being part of the kink community. On a personal level, I had recovered from a terrible breakup and was settling into a new owner-slave dynamic with Faith, a wonderful young male masochist and submissive, as well as training Anna, a young woman whom we determined was more a service dominant than a submissive because she was more comfortable taking the lead but primarily concerned with her partner's desires not her own. I had also released my third book of short stories and had done a few public readings and book signings right in town. I was feeling confident, secure, and happy.

I was not looking for another submissive, and definitely not another slave.

After missing the first month of Headspace meetings in the new semester, Faith and our vice president both said they had something important to tell me. They said they'd met this great, polite, very knowledgeable male top at the last munch and asked if I would please help them encourage him to stay active in the group. This conversation, with two different people at two different times, suggested to me that we might have a wonderful new member for our community. Since community was important to me at that time, I made a point of going to the next workshop after German class, even though I was tired.

I wasn't sure who he was. There were two new young men and two young women (who were practically hanging off one of the young men) at that meeting, plus some of the regulars and semi-regulars. The event was ending soon after I arrived, and Faith came up to me and whispered that that lone young man was the one he'd told me about. I curbed my need to just get home and smiled when Fox introduced himself. He was eager to learn if there was anything scheduled that evening and was clearly disappointed when I said no, the workshops were all we did these evenings, plus I needed to get home after German.

Now, I've literally had young women and some men ask if it's okay for them to "look at Fox," and I've seen his good looks draw shy attention. But to be honest, I don't remember being bowled over by his looks. Instead I was intrigued by his words, his tone of voice and his body language. After wishing him goodnight and reminding him of the Saturday munch, I left with Faith —

whispering to him that he was incorrect; that Fox was not a top. Did I know that? No, I didn't know that. I felt it; I pieced it together, but although I wanted it to be that way, and although I had yet to be incorrect about such an assessment about someone I'd just met, I knew better than to assume. I planned to ask him the next time I saw him.

That would be the Saturday munch. Faith took me to get my hair cut, and I dressed up a bit to make an impression. I sat in the middle of the table where I could mingle better. Soon after we arrived, Fox came in and sat across from me after asking if the seat was taken. This gave us the opportunity to talk more directly. I learned several cool things about him including an interest in role-playing games (I told him about our gaming group), a common mental health issue (a topic we'll cover later in the book), and his major (physics, the same as Tom's in college and grad school). Most importantly, sitting across from him allowed me to observe how he interacted with everyone. He was polite, he was a gentleman, and yes, it was clear he had a lot of knowledge about and interest in bondage. (I do not believe that knowledge equals role, by the way, but I think that is a very common assumption.) He mentioned he'd walked all the way from campus, which was at least three miles. Tom and I offered to give him a lift back to campus, and when he agreed I took the opportunity to ask him what his BDSM orientation was. Submissive, he said.

I have no idea what got into me. I used, or more accurately misused, my position on the steering committee to get his e-mail address, and I messaged him to say what a pleasure it had been to meet him.

He replied and added this flirty little signature to it: "Fox Wolfe, A wolf who can walk by his owner's side without a leash, but what fun is there in that?"

Again, what possessed me? I flirted right back! "So do you have one? An owner, I mean?"

That's how we began. I wasn't looking for someone, but soon we were talking and hanging out, and he was coming to the gaming group. I can't remember now if I encouraged him to apply for training or how that started, but by the middle of October we were in a signed contractual trainer-trainee relationship approved of by Tom, Faith and Anna. That began the busiest few months of my life in terms of being poly. They were also the months that taught me that I really, really wanted a poly, kinky family and taught me that three submissive or slave partners plus a husband is probably the upper limit for me in terms of how many I can have in such a family. A woman still needs time for herself and her career, after all.

Fox remembers: By the spring of my senior year of high school, I had been accepted into two of the three colleges I had applied to. It was a close call, but in the end I chose Bloomington because I was familiar with the campus and it was in-state, had a well-recognized physics program, and had offered me a good scholarship. At 19 years old, I was excited to be on my own and eager to demonstrate to my parents and myself that I could be a responsible, independent adult. I was also eager to attend classes and study all the subjects I'd ever been interested in without the pressures of family and what I regarded as the frustrating social conventions of high school. At least two of the interests I intended to explore more deeply with my newfound freedom, however, were not academic.

As mentioned earlier, I had been searching out information and experience involving BDSM from an early age, but I had been largely limited to psychological texts, a handful of nonfiction written by actual practitioners, online newsgroups/forums, and a single enlightening club scene experience. When I learned that the university had an organized BDSM group open to both students and members of the greater BDSM community, I was absolutely floored! Headspace had been listed in the brochures I had picked up from the GLBT table during orientation, but it had contained little more than a basic description — no mention of scheduled meetings. It wasn't until one evening when I was leaving the dining hall that I happened across a small, locally published newspaper called The Quiver that I saw an ad for an actual Headspace event. It was an erotic book reading being given by an author named TammyJo Eckhart. Sadly, I discovered that The Quiver was published on a monthly basis and I had missed the event by more than a week. The silver lining was that the ad mentioned in tiny print that Headspace met on the first Saturday and every third and fourth Thursday of the month. I was determined to make the Thursday munch. The first thing I did was e-mail the group's steering committee to confirm the time and location. Within 24 hours, I had been contacted by a gentleman called Faith and added to the announcement list.

When Thursday finally came around, I dressed in my best shirt and slacks and walked the three miles from my dorm room across town to the Encore Café. I felt quite nervous but did my best to hide it as I scanned the venue for any sign of overt kinkiness. Thankfully a small, folded cardstock sign with "Headspace" written on it adorned a table with three friendly-looking people seated at it. The first to greet me was a robust man with thick glasses and a winning smile. He was the Faith who'd answered my e-mail (and, as I'd learn later, one of TammyJo's current slaves). The other couple at the table turned out to be the ones responsible for publishing The Quiver. At my core, this is really all I'd been hoping for — simply to be in the company of others who could understand, who shared similar interests and could discuss them openly, and who wouldn't judge me for being kinky.

As the new face at the table, I was the subject of early conversation. I wanted to make a good impression, so I fell back on the manners I'd been raised with and did my best to keep my nervousness from making me hyper. Fortunately, I didn't have to worry about it for very long. The laid-back and easygoing atmosphere (along with a slice of grasshopper pie) soon had me feeling at ease. I felt my nervous energy gradually evaporate as I fielded questions and asked many in return. When the subject of bondage came up, however, they appeared surprised by my level of experience. While a few had done bondage, most were more into sensation play. I found this slightly disappointing, as I had hoped to find someone even more experienced to converse with, but the more I heard, the more confident I became that I'd find such an individual through the group eventually. This led to my inquiring what the next workshop would feature and mentioning the book reading I was sorry to have missed. At that point, they looked at each other and told me I should really meet TammyJo sometime.

Another week passed, and I was waiting in the classroom where the workshop would take place. As would be my habit that first year, I was about ten minutes early. The first ones to arrive were the three I'd met previously, followed soon after by a gentleman and two ladies about my age who sat together beside me. Finally, TammyJo's husband arrived, and we were introduced. I don't actually remember what my first impression of Tom was, but I imagine I saw him as someone I could be good friends with (our geekiness was obviously compatible).

The workshop itself revolved around making a "pervertible" — namely, a flogger composed of a foam-noodle pool toy and a length of garden hose (ridiculous looking, but producing a surprisingly satisfying thud). Near the very end of the workshop, the door to the classroom opened, and a pretty, curly-haired redhead entered and sat beside Tom. She quickly apologized, mentioning a German class which had run late. When the workshop finished, people started chatting about their days and recent activities. It was clear that aside from the trio and myself, these folks were friends even outside the auspices of Headspace, a fact that made me even more eager to belong.

I suppose that's what made me stop TammyJo and Tom as they were leaving so that I could introduce myself. My recollection of the encounter is that it was polite, but very brief (I would learn later on that TammyJo was simply exhausted from her class and wanted to get home). In the end, she simply welcomed me to the group and reminded me of the upcoming Saturday munch. Strangely, I remember being very disappointed that there would be no opportunity to socialize with her until then. One must imagine that I had been attracted on some level at first sight, but whatever the reason I walked home alone that night with a lot on my mind.

The Saturday munch fell on a sunny and hot fall afternoon. Bloomington had been experiencing something of a drought/heat wave and temperatures were still hovering around 95°F. Despite a month of acclimating to the area, I was still wary of the bus system (which I had found to be expensive and frustratingly unreliable), so I walked the three miles from my campus dorm room to the restaurant, Cassidy's. Needless to say, I was greatly relieved to stumble past the curtain of conditioned air. When I finally opened my eyes, I was surprised by a TammyJo entirely different from the one I'd met before. Wearing a long, slim black dress with a red pattern along the hem, the cheerful redhead seemed to float around the table visiting with people before coming to rest beside Tom, who was seated at the far end.

I remember taking a seat on the opposite side and immediately engaging in conversation. TammyJo revealed that she was a teacher at the University working on her doctorate in Ancient History — which was of interest to me because I'd been fascinated since grade school by the works, religion, and funerary rituals of the ancient Egyptians. TammyJo's focus was more on the Greeks and Romans, but she was very well versed in all of Western Civ and happily discussed where my interest in the Egyptians and her specialty overlapped. When she mentioned that her dissertation involved Amazons, however, I had a hard time suppressing my grin. After chatting for even a short while, the idea of a such a strong, dominant woman dedicating herself to the research of the mythology surrounding an ancient matriarchal culture of woman warriors struck me as perfect.

When I was encouraged to talk about myself, I mentioned that I was majoring in physics and had a long-time love of science fiction. This caught the attention of Tom, who held a master's degree in physics and was profoundly well-read.

When the munch finally began to wind down, TammyJo offered me a lift home, which I gladly accepted. As we were leaving, TammyJo turned to ask me what my D/s orientation was. When I answered that I believed myself to be submissive, she mentioned how the others had believed that I was a dominant. This confused me, as I was almost certain I had mentioned my orientation during that first munch at Encore. Had I projected an aura I wasn't aware of? In retrospect, I may have, given that I now consider myself a switch, but Mistress thinks it was because that having knowledge is more often viewed as part of the dominant's role than it is the submissive's.

In any case, it wasn't long before I checked my e-mail and found a message from TammyJo. She did, in fact, mention that she'd used her position to acquire my e-mail from the group mailing list, but I assured her in my reply that I didn't mind. I also mentioned how I enjoyed myself at the munch and looked forward to playing in her RPG as well as taking her up on the offer to peruse her BDSM library. I don't know if I was actually trying to flirt in my reply. I believe at the time I just meant it to be funny, but it opened the door to our relationship.

TammyJo speaks: The first few years are the hardest. As you can tell from our memories of finding each other, we weren't planning on doing much more than getting to know each other. But I already had a small local reputation of being a safe person to explore BDSM with, and while we can't remember the details of how Fox began training, we know he must have filled out my application before it started. It started as my training of Anna did, a way to help someone fairly new to the community learn a wide range of information about being a submissive or slave so that they could determine if that was something they wanted to pursue later on. Most of the time, the people who came to me didn't stay with me; I was used to that and had an almost parental or instructor-like sense of pride when I learned that one of my trainees had been doing well — perhaps one had become very involved in his local community, or another had found herself a good partner.

Training went normally for a while, but fairly soon Fox started developing a deeper emotional connection to me, going so far as to tell me he thought he was falling in love with me one evening. That was a shock to me, because in my entire life, I'd almost always been the one to say those words first. Fox was taking this training thing as a session-by-session experience, though he put as much work into it as Faith ever did. The sad fact was that I didn't feel that way, and I couldn't lie to him, but I did say that I could see myself falling in love with him. That threatened the entire way that training usually went, and yet we didn't stop.

The formal four months of training expanded for Fox into about eight months as he finished his first year of college. During the second half of this training period we found it increasingly difficult to leave scenespace or D/s mentally. We don't know who started being unable to snap out of that mindset when the training collar came off, but it began a feedback loop with one of us saying or doing something that triggered our psychological and emotional conditions that were supposed to be kept to those scheduled training periods. You can control your actions, but your emotions are another matter, and when the reactions you get seem positive and empowering, it is easy to just go with it. We suspect that this flow of authority, this feeling that you just are the dominant or the submissive with this one person, happens to a lot of people. We worked at trying to keep things separated, at making sure we remained equals, as often as we could.

Then that first summer came, and Fox needed a place to live. While he lived on campus, when we only saw each other on weekends or a few days on campus during the week, it was feasible to keep our growing D/s dynamic controlled. Moving in together would change that, and we had a choice to make. We chose to formalize our relationship and signed our first owner-slave contract. We don't recall that first summer being very difficult overall. Things seemed to flow smoothly most of the time. Perhaps it was the newness of the relationship and the ease in which all four of us in the household got along, until Faith took a job in another state too far away to make a continued M/s dynamic rewarding for me. We'll talk more about the specific difficulties and rewards in a poly household, but this was when Fox's duties as a slave started to take on the full spectrum of service.

In the fall, Fox moved out for financial reasons. Taking a job on campus as a resident assistant saved him a lot of money on housing and allowed him to exercise those leadership qualities his parents instilled in him. However, it took him away from me at a time when I was finishing my course work and preparing for my final exams. This is when our first serious challenges began. While both of us were busy, we had grown accustomed to being together a good deal of the time, and for me this created a huge emotional expectation that didn't reflect the current situation.

That year was rough. Fox spent as much free time as he could at the house, and I saw him as often as we could both be on campus. Out of the blue it seemed that something would happen or be said that set one of us off, and as you may have experienced yourselves, this created a hostile situation. Things got so intense at one point that Tom threatened to handcuff us together until we worked this out. For example, we struggled to find time together, but this constantly conflicted with Fox's duties as a resident hall assistant, which was helping to cover the costs of his room and board. We both wanted this relationship, and we had seen how well it could work, so we made the choice and Fox made the sacrifice to move back to the house for good. It was amazing the difference sharing a home made for us, but it wasn't the end of our first few years' struggles.

The next big challenge to our relationship began with a book.[2] I was sent a book to review for my work at that time with KinkyBooks.com, a company that used to do the convention circuit and sell books online but which has been in hiatus for a few years now. I found that the section on natural dominants resonated for me, and I wondered if the corresponding section on natural submissives would ring true for Fox. It did and it didn't. This gave Fox the opportunity to express his dislike of the term "slave," but for me this revelation came as something of a surprise. For a year he had seemingly been happy to answer and identify with that term, and now he actively tried to reject it.

From time to time we hear of other couples and households who face periods of rebellion. When that happens you have to try to find the core of the problem. Fox insisted that he wanted things to stay as they were between us, and yet the word "slave" was repulsive to him. For me that term meant everything: it was the height of devotion and service; it was well beyond what any mere bottom or submissive could be. There will be times in your relationship where one of you will need to make sacrifices; often these fall primarily on the slave, but even when the challenge is a deal-breaker the owner must make the effort to convince and not bully their partner into accepting their way. I probably did a bit of both bullying and convincing, and the result after months of discussion was that Fox became my slave, not a slave.

We faced other challenges in the early years. Fox's family was exceedingly uncomfortable with his living here, and he was unable to fully disclose our dynamic to anyone other than his sister, who was also uncomfortable. Health problems and injuries made us feel less dominant or submissive, as did work and school. We'll cover all these issues in the rest of the book, using ourselves as examples of how to (or how not to) deal with these problems.

The greatest challenge came from two fronts. The first started as Fox neared graduation and had its roots in my history of, and consequent fear of, being abandoned, a fear that I can still feel today. A number of people, a rather shockingly large number of people in fact, began to tell me that Fox would leave as soon as he got that bachelor's degree, and these people came from our local kink community, our vanilla friends, and even Fox's family. We have no idea

---

2   F.R.R. Mallory, *Extreme Space: The Domination and Submission Handbook* (Rohnert Park: Unbound Books, 1998).

why people told me these things. Did they think they were protecting me? We do know why Fox's family expected him to move on — he was finished with school, so of course he would start a career and move away. The result was that I started to actively try to push Fox away.

Don't let anyone tell you that being a slave means being passive. During those months Fox worked hard to show me that his commitment to our relationship was solid, that his promises to serve were not going to be discarded. When his graduation day came and he returned home to our house, that was when it finally hit us that this was potentially for life. That realization solidified our bond, and since then the challenges we've had to our dynamic have been minor ones, the more mundane and vanilla type, which we'll discuss later in this book.

The truth is that there is no simple plan you can follow to make M/s work for you. There is no universal rulebook and no single method that will help you both find happiness in slavery or ownership. What we hope our brief personal history and the rest of this book can do is offer you honest examples of how life can challenge you and how you can purposely create your relationship to withstand any complication. While some of this is specific to dominant women and submissive men, we believe our story and our advice will be helpful to anyone as they begin this journey.

4

MAKING M/s WORK EVERY DAY

Basic Ideas Before You Start

We already dropped one bombshell on you about this idea of power exchange being an inaccurate way of looking at D/s and M/s, but before we get into the nitty-gritty about how to make this all work for your relationship, we want to share a few more ideas about authority-based relationships that may sound radical to some of you. While we aren't claiming any "one true way," we have found these truths in our own journeys. We believe that adjusting how you look at M/s and D/s just a bit may increase your ability to embrace your own identity, find a worthy partner (or partners), and create a life together.

Getting Past the Search for "The One"

Throughout chat rooms and online forums, and at munches around the world, people talk romantically about finding "The One." Aside from the fact that this is really nothing more than the vanilla world's familiar romantic notions about finding one's soulmate, this obsession with finding the one that was made for you does not reflect reality for the vast majority of BDSMers, let alone those in M/s or D/s relationships.

Let's be honest with each other. That rush of adrenaline, the images of your lover in your mind almost constantly, that feeling of connection — all of those are part of the feelings of new love. You've felt it over and over throughout your lifetime, even though bad breakups and sad endings may have hidden it from your conscious mind. It's chemistry, it's biology, and it's something everyone feels when they fall in love in that romantic or erotic sense. So the idea that your feelings will guide you to a single person whom you should be with forever isn't very likely.

Think a bit further: out of billions of people, there is only one for you? What a horrible thought! What if they died last year? What if they married the "wrong" person? What if they live in the mountains of Nepal? What if a car repair prevented you from attending last week's munch, and that was the only time your one true love was going to be at the same location as you? The very idea that you are doomed to be alone seems rather self-defeating to us — not to mention depressing.

Buying into this romantic limitation can be negative on a wide range of levels. When a relationship falls apart (and at least one almost inevitably will at some point in your BDSM journey), you'll be tempted to give up entirely if you think that was your shot at "The One" and you failed. Or even worse, you'll start doubting your judgment and ability to spot a potential partner at all. We've both had these feelings; we aren't just talking theory here. The worst danger in thinking this is your "One" is that it may blind you to an unhealthy and damaging relationship.

If you think that being a slave means you just have to take whatever your owner dishes out, think about how your life impacts others. If you are unhealthy, if you are damaged, you can't really be of service or aid to anyone else, be it a child, your workplace, or even your owner. If you can't give your best, how are you being a good slave? The same is true for owners as well, though it is less common to hear about the dominant being abused in a relationship. Thinking this is "The One" becomes an excuse to let your own life deteriorate. That is not what we want for anyone.

Isn't it better to give yourself hope by thinking of all those billions of people as potential partners to start with, and then using your expectations, personality, location, background, and other criteria to narrow that horde down to a manageable level? We strongly believe that the attitude where you have many potential matches is a much healthier approach to BDSM and to life in general.

Focus on what you have in common with others and what you can learn from others, and allow yourself to take a few risks to find out if that potential partner is more than just another of these billions of people. Much of our relationship's creation revolved around having a wide range of experiences, sometimes from multiple sources and sometimes with multiple people. That isn't the same as having no standards or taking on all comers at the dungeon or during the munch. Never assume that person you are talking to is "The One" or

"The No Way in Hell," either. Let yourself be selectively open to the possibilities, and give up the vanilla concept of "The One" for you.

Easier said than done, huh? Not if you start with yourself. In general, always look in the mirror before you begin your search for a relationship or when your dynamic has a problem. A good deal of the time, the problem begins and may even end with the person reflected back.

Personal Expectations at the Beginning

One way that you set up the criteria for who may be a potential partner is to look at your expectations. Fox likes to claim that he had none when he met TammyJo and that he has none now. What he is probably really trying to say is that he lets himself be open to what might happen and keeps his expectations realistic and probable.

Realistic and Probable.

Make that a mantra for yourself and your relationship. This one change in how you look at M/s and femdom in general may be the most important change you can ever make in your life. By making this adjustment in how you think, you increase your chances of creating a successful long-term relationship — heck, of even finding a potential partner at all.

Let us be clear: fantasies are great! As we'll discuss in our section about "love," fantasy is likely what drew you to BDSM in the first place. But, unless you are enacting a role-playing scenario, writing a story, or acting in a play, you must separate fantasy from reality in order to get your dynamic to work day in and day out.

If you are looking for a 24/7 or M/s dynamic, this probably means you will live together at some point. While relationships of this nature can exist when the people live in different locations, most successful M/s relationships we know about share a domicile. This means you are going to see your partner ill, dressed to deal with the trash, grubbing around outdoors, and interacting with neighbors, family and friends whose knowledge about BDSM is limited or wrong. It is also highly unlikely that you will have the money to live in a mansion and be able to dedicate every hour of your day to achieving kinky fantasy fulfillment.

We'll talk more about Needs and Wants later, but for now, focus on what is Realistic and Probable for you alone. Ask yourself some basic questions. What is your income? Education? Political belief? Your situation with family and friends? How do you honestly feel about yourself?

If you are struggling or find something lacking in any of these areas, how likely are you to attract someone who has it all down perfectly? Not too. While it might be possible that hot starlet or that award-winning hunk might find you attractive and sweep you off your feet, it isn't probable unless you become someone whom they would interact with on a regular basis. Instead of setting your sights on someone out of your circle, look at your life and classify your potential partners from similar backgrounds, interests, and location.

You are most likely to have things in common with someone of a similar economic and cultural background. This doesn't mean you have to be identical (in fact, that could be a bit boring after a while), but you should look for several commonalities. TammyJo's childhood was part of a working-class family in the Midwest, in a religious but practical household. Fox's childhood was part of a more middle-class Midwest background, with religious variations but very practical, too. Both had high expectations placed on them to succeed as children. Both were raised in a Christian tradition, but not with an evangelical or overly conservative dogma. Both had attractions to the arts and to analytical thinking, though they expressed that in different fields when they each went to college. Both knew the sacrifices that their parents had made for their children and this knowledge influenced their high expectations for themselves in college and in life. Both had a sense of duty and honor that they applied to themselves and then to others they interacted with.

So you see — we had several differences, but a lot of commonalities as well. Our similar backgrounds gave us a common place to begin our discussions as well as similar solutions and support when life happens. The differences help us push each other to become better and keep the conversations and activities interesting. Looking within your existing social circles and searching for common interests beyond the latex outfit at a party is a great way to find a potential partner. In other words, set your expectations for who your slave or owner could be within the realm of people you are likely to interact with. You may not need to look overseas or across the country if you get involved in all your nearby communities have to offer. If you ever feel like you have to look far away and settle for a long distance relationship, that is a reflection more of your expectations and willingness to get involved in the kinky community near you than of the reality of how very unique you are — or of how many fakes there are out there.

Of course, you are unique, just like everyone else is — which means your problem finding a partner is all too common. If so many people are looking and complaining about not finding someone, either large numbers of you are blind, because you are ignoring each other, or you simply aren't looking in the best places, and that may be a result of your expectations being unrealistic for you. Stop looking for the porn image of the ideal mistress or slave and start looking around at what is available where you are. Start looking in the mirror and be honest about your own strengths and weaknesses before you look for that perfect someone. You are the biggest obstacle to finding your M/s dynamic.

One of the great things about BDSM becoming more visible since TammyJo started exploring is that you can find munches, workshops, and events around the world now, especially in the USA. Even the most conservative Bible Belt state can boast a few different organizations. Obviously, if you want to have an M/s dynamic, you need to find someone with some basic knowledge about BDSM, as well as having that knowledge yourself. While you can try to find that hidden dominant at church or that submissive at your book club, we really think a good place to start is in the kinky community, coupled with looking for those commonalities in background and interest.

Searching in these venues requires three things from you. First, you have to start going to BDSM events regularly so you become known and can get to know others. Becoming known makes it more likely that people with similar interests will be directed to you by others. It also means you'll have ready character references for potential play partners. Both these factors can be tremendous aids in your search — think back on the story of how we found each other. Every single slave that TammyJo has ever had, she met via a munch or group in her community. People she knew via online ads or forums who refused to get involved generally didn't make it past a few conversations and never past a scene or two.

Second, finding a compatible partner requires that you have conversations that aren't just focused on BDSM. We aren't saying you need to date in the vanilla sense, but you certainly have to get to know each other before you can jump into a D/s dynamic with any sort of informed negotiation (especially if you want this to last for years and years). A fun scene can be had with a club member at a party after a few exchanges of limits and interests, but that only lasts for that one scene unless you take the time to get to know each other and make plans to do so. If you want someone you can live with 24/7 or who can be of service to you or control you day in and day out, you have to be able to do more than a simple flogging or some bondage. Do you have similar beliefs about things? Do you have similar expectations for where you want to be in your careers or lives five years from now? Do you have the same desire for offspring or pets? Yeah, you can go with the "my way or the highway" philosophy of domination, but that's likely to result in a lot of short relationships or unhappy ones.

Finally, to make all of this work you have to be honest about yourself. We aren't saying that you should tell a stranger you met at a munch your entire life story, but don't claim you have a political view, an income, or a fetish that you don't have just because that hottie mentions it. Take the time to figure out as much about yourself as you can. As silly as it may seem, do some career or personality tests, take some self-help classes, read books about subjects and reflect on different viewpoints. Heck, enlarge your circle of friends and examine how you interact with others. Do you have habits that put people off or attract them? If you are putting people off, are you willing to do the work to change?

A huge part of your search for a partner begins with thinking about your expectations for your own life, those not immediately connected to being an owner or a slave. What sort of job do you want to have? What type of house, condo, apartment, or tent do you want to live in? Do you see yourself in a big city, a small town or out in the countryside? How important are family and friends to you? What about religion or entertainment? How do you like to spend your free time? Do you like being with people or prefer being alone? What kinds of food do you like to eat, and what kinds can't you eat? Do you want children and/or pets? Do you think you'll ever be asked to take care of your parents when they get elderly?

These are just some of the questions to ask, and we know that they seem so mundane, so boring, so — to use a common term in the BDSM community — vanilla. Most of your life is spent dealing with these mundane matters regardless of whether or not you are a slave or a mistress. Bills will have to be paid, food will have to be acquired and prepared, and you'll have to interact with people who haven't got a clue about BDSM, let alone D/s or M/s. So, take a good deal of time to figure out what your life is like and what you want it to be like free from any kinky dynamic. This could take an hour, it could take a week, or it could take longer, but do take the time to consider all of this and even write it down. Having an idea of what you want or think your life will be like is a great help in planning for it and making it happen. That's basic advice any career or relationship consultant will give you.

After you have taken this honest assessment of your life and what you want it to look like before kink, imagine yourself as that owner or slave within that life. If you can't see the two working together or you start feeling like you'll need to make all sorts of sacrifices, you might have unrealistic expectations for how M/s works for most people today. The wonderful thing about consensual slavery, which we'll define in the next subsection, is that it can fit well into almost any life you can imagine, almost any income, and almost any culture, as long as you keep your expectations about what it involves Realistic and Probable.

All this self-reflection, all this talking... Geesh, can't we just move on to the collar and the whips, already? Sure, go ahead and jump in. The effort you put into figuring out if you should even take that step is going to influence your chances for success in life as mistress and slave. The more time you spend finding the best materials to build a foundation before you start building it, the more stable your dynamic will be, just like a house.

The Meaning of Consensual Slavery

Within the online community that many of you may be familiar with, the very definition of "slavery" in regards to M/s or D/s or BDSM is hotly debated. Far too often people turn to dictionaries and encyclopedias without considering that BDSM is about consensual adult relationships — NOT institutional, legal or historical slavery. The very use of the terms "slavery" and "slave" is difficult for many people and an incredible turn-on for others. In this section we're going to give you our working definition of consensual slavery, pulled from our experiences, the BDSM community in general, and TammyJo's knowledge about slavery[1] around the world and across time.

"Slavery" and "slave" have several meanings if you look beyond a grade school definition or simplistic online dictionary. Go ahead, start grabbing your dictionaries and encyclopedias and start comparing all those definitions — all of them, not merely the one you agree with or see first. At the core of all of those definitions is the idea that one person is under or answering to the authority of another person. That could describe a lot of statuses in reality, so really you use this word because it has meaning for you, not because it has a legal or economic meaning.

Since we do not live in a society where slavery is legal, in which we would therefore acquire our submissives or slaves through legal means of slavery, the

---

1 One of TammyJo's subfields for her PhD in history was slavery, a study she keeps up on even outside of academia proper.

use of the terms "slave" or "slavery" is merely a matter of our individual, couple, and household desires manifesting themselves. We use the words because they turn us on or because they reflect the degree of authority one partner has over/from the other. We use the words because it feels right for us, not because it reflects an objective legal reality.

In most of the world today in the 21st century, the alternative would be that we were committing a crime by illegally enslaving someone, and if this were true we would run the risk of losing our own freedom to legal entities by claiming we had literally enslaved someone. How successful do you think you'd be at a consensual owner-slave dynamic if one or both of you were in jail? Just because most of the legal cases we have seen thus far have involved male owners and female slaves within or connected to the BDSM community, this does not mean a male slave or even a female owner might not bring the law to their ex's home. Do you want to be that test case? We don't, because we like our lives together and want to stay together.

"Consensual" is a bit more forward in definition. It means that all parties give their mutual agreement to and willingness to something, illegal or not, recognized by the state or not. The definition revolves around the people or parties doing an activity or being part of a relationship — in other words, for something to be consensual it must involve at least two people.

If you put these two terms together — "consensual slavery" — then you have what we believe is a good working and simple definition for M/s: an agreed-upon authority dynamic that those involved call slavery. Some folks say "erotic slavery" too, but as we'll cover in this book, not all M/s dynamics are erotic or sexual in nature.

Wait! Does this mean that two different relationships that look radically different and function radically differently can still be considered consensual slavery or M/s?

To a degree, yes. However, we do need to look at this definition to offer some guidelines. First, have all the parties agreed to their relationship? If they haven't, it isn't consensual. It may have grown from long drawn-out negotiations or simply mutual expectations, but both people have to consent for it to be consensual; it can't be consensual merely because one was bullied into it or one felt that they couldn't do any better, that they didn't deserve any better, or that God wanted things this way. Ideally, we think these dynamics are most healthy and most likely to last a long time when that consent falls somewhere between planned and unplanned. The planning part we'll talk about in the section on how to set up your dynamic, but the unplanned part comes when you find that you start to relate to each other in a D/s or M/s fashion beyond the periods you negotiated and that those interactions feel "natural" and positive for you both.

Second, do those in question use the term "slavery" or "slave" to describe it? We strongly believe that couples/households must have the right to define themselves first and foremost. While you or we might look at a situation and define it one way, is it really right for us to try to shove our definitions onto others? Would you like it if someone did that to you? No, so don't try to define other people's relationships in this fashion, especially if you want the right to define yourself. Within a dynamic there may be disagreements over which words best describe the relationship, but somewhere in their journey that group has decided to embrace this loaded term.

The most important component in this definition is authority. In all dictionary definitions, a slave is under authority — be it the authority of a legal owner, a drug, a passion, or a personal relationship. The authority in an M/s dynamic may be extreme by most modern standards of marriage and friendship, and even according to others in the BDSM community. Think of authority as the recognized right to make things happen in some fashion (this can include yourself, but is generally exercised with regard to other people). Authority can extend to all aspects of life or merely some parts of it. Authority can and will change over time as your relationship develops and you learn more about each other. Authority can be direct (moving someone's body, for example), indirect (telling them to move), or implicit (your desires are part of the reason they decide to move, even if you aren't there).

Having authority and exercising it are not the same. TammyJo has the authority to decide if Fox takes a job offer in another city, an authority which grew over the course of their relationship. However, unless she felt he was having difficulty making such a decision or he wasn't considering all the facts, she is unlikely to exercise that authority. She could dictate when he can use the bathroom, but she finds that idea tedious and unnecessary, taking too much attention from the things she wants to do in her life most of the time. Still, she does have fun exercising a bit of micromanagement for short durations. The big question here is this: Who has the authority? Both people must agree, or they are clearly not in a consensual slavery dynamic.

The best way to determine if someone is in a consensual slavery dynamic, then, is to ask a few questions. Did they both (all) consent? Do they all use that term? Who has the authority in that relationship? If you and your partner agree, then you are in such a relationship, no matter how you compare to others at the next munch or online.

When it comes right down to it, aren't all these questions about defining words and classifying each other merely a symptom of our forgetting what is most important — each other in this relationship — and worrying about what others might think of us? In a status-conscious society — and most societies are concerned with status — it is hard to escape this measurement of yourself. You are never going to match up with everyone you encounter. No matter how hard you try, someone will be better or richer or sexier than you. Work on getting over that concern so you can focus on what matters: you and your partner.

SLAVE DOES NOT EQUAL SUBMISSIVE

The dominant culture that the BDSM subculture exists within is patriarchal throughout most of the world. Sometimes it is a decaying patriarchy, such as in Europe, but sometimes it thrives, as in the Middle East. Yet take a look at all the online communities, and you'll find men from all over the world claiming to be submissive, looking for that woman to own them. Look at the number of professional dominants who can charge hundreds of dollars for a few hours, and you can see that a market exists around the world for women exercising some authority over men, even if it is for a short period of time. Regardless of whether or not these practitioners' definitions of submissive match each other, this phenomenon suggests that the dominant culture has failed to convince all men that they must remain on top at all times, and it has allowed some women to experience the responsibilities and privileges of authority.

Unfortunately, men who are attracted to submission and service are still products of their cultures. These cultures by and large preach that men should be dominant or at least equals to their partners, serving only a higher authority such as a deity or a military official — rarely if ever a woman. It isn't surprising, then, if a man struggles with some conflict over his desires, be they limited to the bedroom or expanded to a 24/7 life. We want to address one of the big claims about being a slave that can heavily conflict with a man's identity: the idea that being a slave means being submissive.

Submission is often seen as a feminine quality, and having feminine qualities is still frowned upon for most men around the world. Submission is often viewed as doing what you are told, following instructions and putting your own needs and desires after those of the person dominating you. In a sense submission is often seen as being a sort of puppet that the dominant controls. As a man you aren't supposed to be anyone's puppet, particularly not a woman's.

Women have made progress in the decaying patriarchies and even in some actual patriarchies. Increasingly, they can get an education — a privilege once limited to men — or hold jobs once seen as men's positions. Even in terms of clothing or behavior, being masculine is seen as more positive for both men and women, but being feminine is only positive for women. Of course, you can still find religious groups preaching that women should submit to their husbands, but often when you look at their lives you notice women holding down jobs and making decisions, and certainly not waiting around for orders.

This can have an huge impact on a man. As Fox has sometimes expressed, the social expectations are far more limited for men from the man's point of view, especially if you display any tendencies associated too strongly with being a woman. Sometimes it feels as if even doing those traditionally masculine things such as becoming a doctor and providing for a family isn't enough to prove you are a man. It's something you are constantly obligated to prove to anyone who might be judging you. If you are a male, Fox's feelings may sound similar to your own. If you are a woman reading this, these ideas might surprise you, but yes, they too are constantly being judged by the world around them on whether they are man enough.

This is a matter of gender differing from sex, or social expectations differing from biology. Masculine and feminine are genders, male and female are sexes, and there has never been an absolutely one-to-one correlation between sex and gender at any point in human history of which we are aware. It is and has been common throughout the world for individual men and women to reject their gender roles or to push their boundaries. Usually this involves paying a price that many of us would be afraid of, unless that culture has a set aside a third or fourth gender.

Why is this a problem at all in an alternative subculture like BDSM? Shouldn't we have tossed these mundane, vanilla ideas out? Time and again you see from the online gurus that submissive and slave go hand in hand. Some even claim that you must be 100% submissive all the time to be a "real slave." This claim is fed by hundreds of slaves proclaiming they are micromanaged all the time and never have a thought of their own, all the while paradoxically typing away on a forum or a blog. Or perhaps they claim to be kept naked and chained in a cage, unable to even use the toilet without an owner's consent, again with the mysterious computer access. You can still see hundreds of believers in male superiority out there claiming that being a slave or being submissive is being a woman, being feminine, and any man who wants that isn't a "real" man.

To make things even more difficult, if you believe a lot of the hype in the mainstream media and some of the stuff on the Internet, you'd equate being submissive with being passive. Perhaps men are not supposed to be submissive to anyone but those in much higher authority, but even when they are submitting to God or their commanding officer, they certainly are not supposed to be passive, because they have a job to do — they must actively serve their leader. For thousands of years in the Western world, passivity has been equated with weakness, inability, and incompetence. Passivity is rarely seen as a positive feminine trait either. When discussing sexual intercourse, the ancient Greeks, one of the most patriarchal societies in history, might have classified the penetrator as the active partner and the one penetrated as the passive partner, but they also expected wives to be able to run efficient households, oversee slaves, and raise children, all while playing an active role in the religious welfare of the entire city-state; this is hardly being passive. Indeed, ancient Greek women were portrayed as very active in their families and communities, just not in the same way as men. So, equating passive with submissive places a person with those feelings even lower down the scale of social status. How much further from masculine can one get if not even women are supposed to be passive?

Talk about a hard road to walk. Submissive men, men who desire to serve as consensual slaves, are on one of the most difficult journeys in the world today, because they have rejected patriarchal privilege and embraced their own heart's calling instead.

Wait. Couldn't we say that's actually being a good man? Standing up for yourself, refusing to follow the herd? We could, and we do indeed say this, but it just isn't making it through to a lot of submissive men and dominant women out there, because they are trapped by their concepts of gender and their ideas of what slavery entails.

We're going to get a bit geeky here and talk about how legal slavery worked in historical slave-owning societies, how we've noticed consensual slavery working between couples and within households in the modern world, and how it works for us. By the end we hope you will see that slave does not equal submissive all of the time.

In historical slave-owning societies, slaves served two primary functions. The first was economic: they were there to increase the owner's holdings or to help maintain the holdings without being a material burden on the owner. This meant that the work a slave did had to at least equal the cost of feeding, clothing, and sheltering them. Ideally, a slave contributed more, so that the owner's family could enjoy more leisure time and more luxury. While individual slaves might have had their time seriously micromanaged, most owners did not have the desire or time to do that and left it to higher-ranking slaves. This means that from an economic viewpoint, not only did some slaves have to be active, but some had to have authority to make decisions and determine what needed to be done. They couldn't be submissive or passive at all times, just waiting around for orders.

The other function slaves served in such societies was one of displaying an owner's status, along with land, livestock, luxury items, and political power. An owner's status was partly demonstrated by how many slaves he or she had, that's true, but it was also shown by how well those slaves worked and in which jobs. An owner who had to constantly give instructions during a dinner party would be seen as ineffective at best. An owner who couldn't participate in the world of his fellow citizens because he had to oversee the daily lives of his slaves was viewed as a fool. An owner who had to instruct her slaves on daily assignments and be there to make sure they were done would be a failure as a wife and mother because she would not have time to care for her husband or children adequately. Yes, women have been slave owners throughout time and in their own right, not merely as substitutes for their husbands or fathers, so you have historical models out there, ladies.

In a slave-owning society, being a respected slave owner wasn't about owning so much as having a functioning staff that did the work so you could benefit with little direct control from you. Being a good slave was doing what was required, knowing your job and doing it on a consistent basis, and not drawing unnecessary attention to yourself. If you think about the roles of owner and slave this way, the owner might be objectively viewed as more passive and the slave as more active.

As for submission in slave-owning societies, submission was legal and idealized as part of being a good slave. But it wasn't expected, if you look at all the advice given between slave owners and written into legal codes. Slaves were seen as liars and thieves, wily creatures who would rob you of their labor and their bodies at a moment's chance. A good owner kept his slaves in fear of his authority so they didn't step out of line. A good owner watched the household supplies so she'd know when things went missing. In other words, the owners macromanaged their holdings, setting up a system to make things function, placing the rare trustworthy slaves in charge and then turning to society and its laws and customs to dictate to everyone that this was how things must work.

In summary: even in "real slavery," no slave was submissive or passive 100% of the time.

Now back to modern times — within BDSM, there are several different groups who have different styles and ideas about relationships. Those of us who do M/s or 24/7 D/s dynamics are actually in the minority, regardless of what you may have seen on Internet forums or porn sites. We have been privileged to get to know a few other consensual-slavery couples and households over the years, and what we see in our own relationships is often reflective of what we've seen in those that have also lasted for years. We can't speak to what goes on privately beyond that which has been shared with us and what we've observed, but this is our understanding of what is happening in those relationships.

- *The owner has the top level of authority and is viewed as in charge by everyone in that household.*
- *There are degrees of authority given to slaves within the household.*
- *Slaves are expected to communicate clearly about their needs.*
- *Slaves are expected to do their duties independently with minimum oversight from the owner and perform them to the best of their ability.*
- *Slaves are expected to be obedient to any orders from the owner.*
- *Owners are expected to take into consideration information given to them by everyone.*
- *Often there is time set aside to evaluate how things are working.*

This is a simplified view of how these relationships work. For now, do you notice how active each member of the dynamic must be? Do you notice that the owner does not burden herself with making every decision on a daily basis? Do you notice how they all work together to make things function?

On an emotional level we also notice that within these long-term D/s and M/s dynamics there are a lot of positive feelings toward each other and toward the self. Both owners and slaves feel like they are expressing parts of themselves, and that this helps make them happier, perhaps even better, people. When you talk to these couples and families, what you hear is the respect they have for each other and for the work each does to make things function. You might also notice that the slave is not as submissive as porn would lead you to believe — joking and teasing the owner, making decisions, and interacting with others, while at the same time being attentive to the owner and obedient to any of her commands.

Some M/s dynamics are heavily structured with rules and rituals (what we call protocols), while others are more laid back. We'll talk more about what you will need to do to set things up and keep things going later, but for now just understand that no two dynamics look the same or function in quite the same way. In all of them, the work to maintain the relationship is shared, and that means that no one can be passive or submissive all the time.

That should be good news for you submissive men out there. You don't have to give up your manhood or be less masculine to serve. You just need to find ways to balance what you've been taught with what you desire. If you still struggle with the idea that you should never submit to someone unless they are a higher authority than you, guess what? Your mistress is that higher authority, because you have both agreed she is. You fulfill your masculine role as protector and as self-sufficient by serving another, just as you would through military or religious service. I doubt you're going to tell a Marine that he is a wimp, so try to stop seeing yourself as less of a man for having these desires.

In fact, there are several positive role models that submissive men and male slaves can turn to for inspiration. The men below serve someone in authority over them, male or female, without sacrificing their masculinity and often seen as enhancing it through such service:

- *Soldier*
- *Priest*
- *Knight*
- *Bodyguard*
- *Majordomo*

These are just a few. Take some time and try to come up with your own list of men who serve others. What do they have in common? How are these roles masculine? How are they examples of service or submission? How do you feel about taking on a similar role in a relationship?

It could be that some of you reading this want to reject the masculine role or some of the pressure that comes with being a man. That's fine, too, but TammyJo and Fox can't really speak very well to those types of dynamics and what makes them succeed in the long term.

We can say that both on the Internet and offline, one of the biggest complaints we've seen from dominant women is the lack of men who want to be submissive or go that further step into consensual slavery. We don't think they mean a shortage of males in terms of biology, but those who are masculine in terms of gender or gender identity. They mean submissives who are undeniably masculine in all the positive ways and not in the stereotyped negative ways. They're looking for the guy who will stand up for them if need be, who will carry heavy things or get that package down from the high shelf, who can hold down a good job and help support the family, one who looks like a man in all ways but just does it on his knees and obeying her commands. You might think of this as an extreme form of chivalry, and few things are as masculine as chivalry.

If you think you have to be less of a man or submissive all the time if you're going to be a slave, we're telling you that you don't. You really, really don't.

The Role of "Love"

Whether or not you must be in love with your owner or whether you can risk loving your slave is a topic we've seen debated online and discussed offline numerous times. In these debates, there tend to be two camps of belief that get the greatest play. The first believes that love is the foundation of any successful BDSM encounter. They'll go on and on about how their submissive is the love of their life or how they eat, drink and breathe their owner. Then you have the folks on the other side, who think that love corrupts the dynamic. They'll argue that any owner who starts to think of the slave's needs and wants more than their own is a fool who will soon become enslaved, and those on the submissive side agree that they could never expect someone who said "I love you" to treat them like the slave they are. Of course there are those of us who think the entire debate is rather polarizing and unnecessary. The fact that these debates keep happening, however, indicates a deep concern about the role of "love" in BDSM.

There are three basic problems that fuel each of these debates. First, there is the assumption that what works for one relationship must be how things must work for all other relationships. Does that work in the vanilla world? Does that work in the business world? Where exactly do you see the fact that how things work for you is how it must work for someone else? TammyJo's a historian, and she has seen quite the opposite throughout history. With his background in psychology, Fox can see basic trends and requirements for the human psyche, but there are no identical minds and no identical therapeutic models that work for everyone. Human beings are too diverse to really be described by a "one model fits all" approach to anything.

The second problem is that in many languages there is a dearth of words to describe "love," which is a very complex human feeling. Many mental health care professionals and pop psychologists turn to Greek to find words to describe different types of love that human beings are capable of, so we'll use those definitions too, for the rest of this section and book. We'll work the definitions of these terms into the discussion of each type's benefits for a owner-slave dynamic in a few paragraphs, but we want to finish talking about the debates first.

The final problem for these "love" debates, a common problem for any debate in BDSM communities, is that words such as "master," "mistress," "slave," "pet," or whatever else you want to choose do not have fixed, universally-recognized meanings. A good deal of these debates lose focus on the topic of "love" and become battlegrounds for arguing about definitions and connotations of words commonly used in the general community. Numerous people decry the lack of some great "book of kink" that codifies everything, but we think the various meanings of the terms reflect both how they are used by different people and how they change over time. Pick up a dictionary. How many words in there have only one meaning? Not many. So why would the words used in BDSM need to have a single meaning? Yes, a single definition would make things clearer, but it also stifles individual expression, and we can't get behind that idea. Better to talk to your partner about all these things and come to an agreement about terms if you can.

These debates about "love" grow out of real situations in D/s and M/s relationships. We've met and talked with dominants who bemoan the fact that since falling in love they just can't do SM anymore with their partner and that the thought of engaging in that humiliation play they both used to enjoy just turns their stomachs. We've encountered submissives that are so enthralled by their partner that they accept anything that is done to them, their property, or their family, all in the name of love, then cry when it isn't returned. In both cases, the people we've talked to are miserable. Their partners tend to be less than thrilled with the situation as well. The result is either continued sorrow in the dynamic or the termination of it. People afflicted with these consequences of falling in "love" seem to us to be separating BDSM from healthy, loving relationships in their minds or buying into the romantic notion that if you give love you will always receive the same amount back, if not more.

Instead we want to talk about the realities of how "love" can work in BDSM relationships for a healthy, long-term dynamic. Remember that we mentioned the various Greek words for love a short while ago? Now we're going to get back to that, along with examples from our lives of how these have been positive forces in our various BDSM relationships — especially of the femdom variety. These come from ancient Greek, but we're going to Anglicize them for your convenience and simplify the definitions. Three of these you have likely encountered before, but the other two also offer interesting insights to love, relationships, and BDSM.

Agápe is a feeling of contentment and respect.

Contentment is developed when you feel that what you are giving to a relationship is at least equal to what you are getting back. Feeling this way is one way that trust is built, and trust seems to be a foundation upon which most positive human relationships are built, whether it is personal, business, political or religious. If you feel your M/s dynamic is a constant struggle to maintain, you are not feeling contentment, and your trust will be eroded over time — your trust in your partner for his being a jerk, or your trust in yourself for allowing the negative situation to happen to you. Contentment, however, can harm an M/s dynamic if one or both is just letting things flow along without thinking about how to maintain the authority difference you've set up. You might wake up one day and realize you are no longer mistress and slave, and that could cause problems.

Respect is a feeling that someone is worthy in some fashion. With all the porn models of "worthless worms" groveling at leather-clad dominatrixes' feet, you might think this doesn't work in the femdom dynamic. But the simple fact is, unless you feel your partner is worthy of it, you will not put in the work needed to set up or maintain your M/s relationship. At the initial stages we offer respect to each other as human beings, but in order for respect to be built it must be earned through keeping your word, making your actions match your words, and consistent behavior. That is true regardless of which side of the M/s equation you fall into. If TammyJo can't trust that Fox will do as commanded or trained, she soon loses respect for his abilities as a slave and as a man. If he can't feel certain she will maintain her rules in a predictable fashion, he'll feel insecure, which erodes both the feelings of contentment and respect.

So *agápe* is very important in setting up and maintaining your relationship because it reflects feelings of safety and security and helps motivate you to do the work necessary to keep the dynamic going. If one party starts to lag in this feeling, the effects will be felt in the relationship at some point, and usually not in a good way.

Éros is a passionate feeling of desire or longing, from which English derives the word "erotic."

Note that this is a feeling, not an action — so equating éros with sex isn't telling the whole story. Something we hope you've noticed so far in your relationship or search for one is that desiring or longing for something can be a powerful force, affecting the decisions you make to send that email or dress a certain way. Éros is probably the force driving most of us to even look into BDSM at all. We saw a picture or read a story that got us wet or hard, that created éros in us, to learn more about what the heck was going on, what this kinky stuff was all about that got you so hot. It may also be a longing for a type of relationship you've heard about or read about that makes you feel attractive, or an attraction toward another or an object. The beginnings of fetishes may also be a result of éros, but we'll talk more about fetishes later.

So this desire, often of a sexual nature, is very common for both men and women looking for BDSM relationships. But "common" does not mean it is identical from one relationship to the next. One stereotype we're sure you've heard is that men want sex far more often than women. This is a stereotype born out of conservative Victorian values, ideals that did not actually reflect the realities of their times, when flagellation brothels were beginning and prostitution was running rampant. These false ideals, which different classes used to make themselves feel superior to others and which religious authorities used to bolster their power, entered American culture as part of the virtues we are supposed to pursue while also reinforcing the idea that males and females are radically different – a belief that helps keep inequality alive in the greater society. The fact is that different people have different sex drives, and these change with age, health, and the general conditions of life, as well as the expectations one was raised with. Éros may draw you and your partner together, and it can fuel some very hot scenes, but it will change over time, usually fading to a degree, though probably not entirely disappearing, unless other parts of your relationship are unhealthy or you are ill. We'll talk more about sex later on as well.

The biggest problem for éros is that it can be seriously imbalanced in your M/s relationship. Note the word "seriously" here. It is very rare that two people will feel the exact same intensity of any type of love, even the éros that usually burns brightest right at the beginning of a relationship. Remember, your owner-slave dynamic takes work from both of you, and if one of you feels seriously less passion from the other, it will decrease either the éros itself or the types of love you may need to feel if this relationship is worth your time and effort. This happened to TammyJo's relationship with Faith, the slave she owned when she was introduced to Fox. It was clear to everyone, her included, that Faith felt a lot of éros toward her. She didn't return those feelings; for some reason they just weren't there for her in regards to him. Ultimately this must have been a factor in his decision to take a job in another city, especially after he saw her passion toward another slave.

For now, realize that éros is a large part of the initial attraction for many of us. It is going to change over time, and it is unlikely to be a strong motivation to do necessary relationship work if you can more easily get a sexual fix from someone else with less work. You can't control what creates this passion in you, but you also shouldn't expect a partner who has those feelings toward you to just accept nothing in exchange. Using your position as slave or owner is an excuse that is beneath anyone mature enough to be thinking of being in a M/s dynamic in the first place.

Philía is a feeling of commonality and mutual interests.

This is the love that makes communities work, groups function, and friendships thrive, even through difficult times and without external rules like the law or religion. This feeling that we have shared goals and interests motivates people to action. It can motivate a couple, a family or a household to focus their collective energies on a goal such as saving money for a home improvement or setting aside time each night to spend time together. Philía is probably the second reason you find yourself drawn to a potential BDSM partner.

Stroge is an affection you feel toward someone because of the relationship.

Think of this as a functional type of love. It exists because you are raised to believe it should, like the love of mother or love of country. It can refer to activities, a love of sports, or organization, a love for the Church. It can be positive or negative, because it is something you are supposed to feel. In a healthy relationship the feelings are positive and support a dynamic that makes you healthier, happier and better. In an unhealthy relationship this stroge becomes the trap you find yourself in that prevents you from taking action to help or protect yourself, such as the love you might feel toward an abusive partner.

In an owner-slave dynamic, both partners should feel stroge toward the dynamic itself. This means that they value the roles, find them healthy, and will do the work necessary to maintain them. Life is going to throw curve balls at you, and if you can make this commitment to the relationship's structure, you will find it easier to keep up most of the aspects of your dynamic, which we'll discuss in the next section. Think of your M/s dynamic as a marriage (which it may or may not be, legally or religiously speaking). For a marriage to succeed, the partners must not only love each other, but also the institution. If they don't, why go to the expense of getting married in the first place? Setting up your mistress-slave relationship is just the same — if you could share your life and be happy without this D/s structure, why set it up at all? Why not just let it fade over time? After all, it would fit far more easily into the society around you if you did that. So you have to value or have stroge toward your dynamic itself and the roles you each hold in it.

Stroge can be used to support a dynamic that lacks other forms of love, but generally this works best if your relationship is recognized by the culture around you in some fashion, because then you have a model or structure to fall back on. Your M/s dynamic is probably not recognized; indeed, it may be reviled by your society, so you have to have this feeling in order to structure it and make it last.

Thélema is the desire or will to do something.

It's a fair question as to whether this is love, as in a feeling, or whether it goes beyond a feeling into action. Think of it as the feeling that pushes you to do something, that goes beyond the other forms of love. You can feel all of those other types of love and just do nothing with the feeling, never share it, never tell another person, just hold it inside. But thélema equals action. As such, of all the types of love you might feel in BDSM, this is the one you need to go beyond the thoughts and fantasies and start living M/s as part of your life.

Never forget that, for all these types of "love," you need to feel love for yourself first and foremost before you can truly feel it toward another person. Otherwise, you risk losing your ability to say "yes" or "no" to anything in your life. That might sound fun in fantasy, but it isn't very healthy for any adult in the long term.

So the short answer is: Yes, you need love to make M/s work.

This love question is particularly important to the last common issue we want to address before we move on to how you set up your M/s femdom relationship. Love has destroyed many a fun, kinky relationship, and we do not want it to ruin yours.

"Hurt" does not Equal "Harm"

For dominants of both sexes, straight, bi, gay or lesbian, transgendered or not, one of the biggest challenges we can face is doing SM or some of the rougher verbal play that we and our partners enjoy. The reason is simple: Most of us are taught not to hurt other people unless we have no choice. This is especially true for women, as any self-defense instructor will confirm, because women are taught to be even less physically aggressive, though you need only spend a few minutes on a playground to see how nasty little and teen girls can get verbally.

TammyJo has tried to comfort dominants and tops who have lost partners because they "fell in love" and couldn't do all of the fun things they used to do before. After talking with them, the reason became fairly clear. While they might proclaim they are sadists, and they might go to the munches and the play parties, deep inside they still believe all that pop culture and psychological jargon about sadism and BDSM. They reason that if they really love their partners, they can't possibly hurt them,. How disappointing to that partner who loves a hearty spanking, nasty teasing, or any number of things that could hurt them in the way they enjoy.

This type of thinking isn't uncommon, especially among new tops and dominants, and particularly for women, but it will continue as the years go by unless you can tackle this mindset. We aren't saying we want you to throw social politeness out the window or become a mean ball-busting bitch in every interaction, but if you can't give your partner the things they enjoy, if you can't continue to do the things you've enjoyed in the past just because you've "fallen in love," then you have a serious problem that may result in ending your relationship or forcing it to become more vanilla than either of you would like.

The first step in figuring out why you think that love equals not hurting your beloved is understanding where that idea came from. Right now, take some time and try to think of all the messages you personally have gotten that tell you this is true. It may take you a while to sort this out, so don't hurry this task. You are working to build a lifetime of domination or submission, and that takes time. Go on, do it; the book will still be here when you finish, whether it is in an hour, a week, or longer.

When you have your list, look at it and decide who or what gave you each message. Now, as an adult woman, what do you think about these messages? Why do you think that source gave you this message? Do you think it reflected that person's own life? How much do you want to reflect their life now? Again this may take some time, but we encourage you to try this exercise.

Set that aside and think about how you feel when you do something to hurt someone consensually. How does it feel to you to wield that flogger? What does it do to your mind and body when you direct that verbal barb? In your mind, change the person you are doing this to from your loved one to another person

— maybe some celebrity you've fantasized about. Do not imagine someone you've had a breakup or a bad relationship with, because you might get off on the revenge aspect. What you are trying to gauge is what you get out of doing that "hurtful stuff" like SM or humiliation. If you don't get anything positive from it, why have you been doing it? If you do get something positive from it, do you really need to give that up just because you've fallen in love?

We don't think so. We think that if you as the dominant enjoy being rough, nasty, or mean, but do it from a place of pleasure for yourself and underlying respect for your partner, these hurtful things can be very healthy to your relationship. The health here is about getting your needs and wants met, because if those aren't met, you and your dynamic are going to suffer in a nonconsensual and unhealthy way.

There is a difference between things that hurt and things that harm. By harm we mean doing damage that will limit or negatively affect yourself or your partner either physically, emotionally, or spiritually. Flogging someone, even flogging them until they get such a high that they need help walking for a bit, is still hurting them, but flogging them until they can't walk on their own for days is harming them. From a purely selfish viewpoint, if you harm your slave he can't serve you in the best fashion, so you are also harming yourself. From a realistic viewpoint, harming someone is very likely to create serious negative feelings that can poison your relationship and risk pushing your partner so far away that you end up losing them entirely. At its worst, harming someone can get you in trouble with the law, and you may find yourself in jail. Never assume that because you are a woman the cops won't take a man's complaint about you seriously. Times have changed, and the authorities may indeed come knocking on your door. For us, harming someone goes against our personal moral and ethical codes.

How do you know where the line is between hurt and harm? With physical sensation it is a matter of finding a good mentor or teacher and learning proper techniques coupled with paying attention to your bottom's reactions. For emotional harm you need to take the time to get to know your partner, learn about his background, and listen to his voice as well as watch his body language when you discuss things like verbal abuse. If he says he's fine with being called worthless but moves slightly away from you when he says it, or looks away, he probably isn't really fine with it; he just thinks he should be accepting of whatever you want. In matters of the spirit we believe you need to respect your partner's religious or spiritual beliefs or lack thereof; making fun of these often deeply held philosophies can be just as damaging as breaking a rib and risks alienating them from you.

You should be able to avoid most harm simply by going slowly, learning all you can, and paying attention to your partner and your own skill level. However, accidents happen, and sometimes accidents can cause harm. Generally this means physical harm, and you can address this by immediately stopping the scene, reassuring each other that you are both OK, or assessing what you need to do to make the physical harm OK, including going to a doctor or a hospital if necessary. Then you take steps to help that physical harm heal. There is a potential here for emotional harm from accidents, but if you immediately admit you made an error and apologize, things should be fine between you two as long as your actions follow your words.

Here's an example from our life. Once during a bondage scene, Fox got very dizzy, and his blood sugar crashed; he started to topple over, and TammyJo didn't do the greatest job of catching him. Luckily, because of experience, we had set up the room so that he couldn't harm his head by hitting it on something, though he did get dizzy and pulled some muscles. TammyJo immediately undid the bondage, pulled him up and made him comfortable while checking in verbally. Then she got him some food and something to drink and sat with him until he was steady. The harm was minimal for Fox and TammyJo both. The end result was that we felt closer after this error than we did before.

But there had been a real danger that this error could have damaged our trust and our relationship. It could have been a disaster — Fox could have been physically harmed, and the event could have shaken TammyJo's confidence to the point of not wanting to do that type of bondage again. How did we avoid that?

First, we set up the room to give us space and had a soft bed right behind Fox so he could fall on it. Second, we let our levels of experience with that type of scene direct how quickly we went. Third, TammyJo kept checking in, and Fox replied until he, well, just couldn't. There are other things we could have done in hindsight — we could have made sure Fox had eaten before the play, and TammyJo could have practiced moving him around when he was immobilized.

Verbal abuse or humiliation is a more tricky matter than physical SM but still falls within the category of activities that can become harmful. One way to avoid harm but still give your partner the intensity they want is to negotiate what words or phrases are off-limits. We'll say it as often as we need to, but: no, giving each other information and setting limits is not topping from the bottom, so work at figuring out what is a turn-on, what is a turn-off, and what may trigger harmful feelings. You'll want to avoid any terms or phrases that have harmed your partner in the past. If your partner has been teased or bullied about his weight, his hair, his voice, and especially his masculinity, you need to look at other things to turn you or him on. He may have issues with some words about his behavior or even his body that make him tense up or stir up negative emotions.

The terms that make one man hard may make another snap in anger or withdraw emotionally. Don't assume; ask, and even after you ask go slowly with humiliation and verbal abuse, and observe body language and verbal responses. A strong and confident mistress is never worried about stopping or changing tactics if she feels things aren't going as she or her slave wants.

The reason you have to go this extra step of slowing down and watching for signs is that men often agree to certain activities because they are thinking more about orgasm or about pleasing you than about what is healthy for themselves. One way to get around that (though not entirely avoid it) is to also ask for information from the potential submissive before you give your own. TammyJo experimented with this technique for several years. She found that by using checklists coupled with discussions she could gather more reliable information than she got simply from having conversations, because she could cover all the wanted categories. However, what she found was that when she gave her own preferences first, the would-be submissive's desires "magically" matched her own to a very high degree. When she reversed that (getting his information first, then sharing hers), she also noticed that the potential partner would try to change his answers to match hers. Nope, she wanted the undoctored answers, and we suspect you too need complete honesty to help you make the best choices.

As in the case of physical SM, verbal abuse and humiliation can accidentally cross the line from hurt to harm in a matter of seconds. If that happens, we advise you to immediately use your own safeword (yes, as a dominant you should have one, too) and end the scene. Notice that we said end the scene, not leave your owner-slave dynamic; there is a difference. Breaking out of the D/s completely can be too jarring for the harmed person, so back off, stop what you are doing, and verbally reassure him that you still want him and that last phrase, term or activity seemed too intense for him. Sit down in a comfortable place, lower your voice to calm you both down, and just be with each other for a while until things have settled. Then you can try to access what happened. Your slave may not know — he may have reacted on a purely gut level, or the activities or words may have triggered memories buried deep inside. Give him space and time to work it out, and just offer him an open invitation for when he can talk.

For the dominant, making an error in the emotional realm of play can be even more damaging that misjudging where to place the next stroke from a flogger or cane. There are several reasons for this. First, as a woman you have probably been brought up with the expectation that you will be able to take care of others and figure out what is going on with someone emotionally. Making this error may cause you to mistrust your own abilities. Furthermore, while a slave harmed by a physical error is often quite eager to reassure you that he is fine, he may not be able to offer such reassurance when the trigger is mental and emotional. You may have to cope alone for quite some time. This is one very good reason to have other dominants or at least good friends who know you are kinky to talk with. You aren't a bad mistress because your slave broke down into uncontrollable tears if you realized what was happening and dealt with it immediately. You aren't unworthy of his devotion simply because you went a bit too fast, as long as you backed off and kept control of the situation. Remember, motivation and your response is what makes SM in all forms a healthy part of your relationship, not the actions or consequences themselves.

Ladies, try things slowly, react as calmly and honestly as you can, and learn from each scene and each interaction with your slave. Ultimately this attitude toward your play, your partner, and your responsibilities will curb any harm you might do and help you enjoy all that wonderful hurting you may both want.

All of this requires that the bottom give reactions and be honest in his assessment about what is happening to his body, mind, and soul — not only when asked, but also if he feels his limits being reached. With a new submissive this is tricky, because his fantasies may be in areas where his experience is limited. We recommend that new submissives invest time in getting to learn all they can about those things they've fantasized about before they jump headfirst into any relationship. Ask your new top or dominant to go slowly, and if she won't or makes fun of you for that request, well, you need to ask whether she's worthy of your service in the first place.

To some of you this probably sounds like "topping from the bottom," and we despise this phrase. Asking them for what you need and want during negotiation, and giving information during a scene, is not "topping from the bottom" at all. It is being open; it is giving the dominant everything, including your thoughts and feelings. "Topping from the bottom" would be dictating how you want the scene to progress or criticizing the flow of things while they are happening. Being submissive means accepting the directions and decisions of another for a period of time. If you move on to becoming a slave, that means accepting those things 24/7. Dominants cannot give directions or make decisions without your information, so refusing to give feedback or express your desires because you worry about "topping from the bottom" is actually refusing to submit.

There is one final issue we need to address in this section on hurt versus harm. Sometimes a sadist is not matched with a masochist, or vice versa. If you recall, we talked about having realistic expectations and finding a great match. Sometimes, you match on so many other things that you decide you can overlook some differences, and one of these can be physical or verbal SM.

If you are not a sadist or are not as heavy sadist as your slave might want, you have a dual obligation that you need to keep in mind. Obviously, as the owner, you have the authority to decide when and how things will happen in your relationship. However, if you want your partner to stick around and you want the best service they can give, you need to give them something in return, and for a masochist this means intense physical or emotional stimulation. There is nothing wrong with your setting limits on what you will and will not do. Dominants have limits, too, because they are just human beings.

TammyJo has dealt with a few unequal relationships, in the sense of having a partner who wanted her to be a heavier sadist than she is. In general, she believes that if she feels neutral about some type of play, she should learn the technique and give it a go every now and again. One way to do this is to schedule heavier play time or use it as a reward. Since she is a reaction sadist (meaning that she feeds off the reactions, not the activity of giving pain or seeing someone in pain), she can give her masochistic partners some smaller level of pain or bondage, or even mild verbal humiliation, on a fairly regular basis. That might scratch the itch, but it won't be what they really want, so she feels it is her duty to herself and her slave to make that time. Spreading out a 2000-stroke flogging session into two weekends accomplished the goal of "ringing in the New Year" while letting her rest and also gave the masochist she owned more days of wonderful pain overall. By putting that scene into the context of a special celebration, they also gave each other a gift that honored each one's desires to support their dynamic.

Fox, who is not a masochist, has also dealt with being in a relationship with a sadist. Again, it is a matter of seeing his role as one of service as a slave and gauging what is neutral for him and what is a limit. By reacting to any painful stimulation, he's learned he can give the sadist in his life the responses she wants, and this satisfies much of what she needs on a regular basis. More intense scenes from time to time then become personal challenges he undertakes to endure for the sake of pleasing her. He also exercises his trust in her by truly suffering, knowing she is going to verbally encourage him and give him necessary aftercare when she's done.

You can make unevenly-matched desires for intense or even hurtful interactions work, but you have to each give and take. You also must make sure you steer clear of harming either one of you, through good communication, honest assessments of what you can and cannot do, and reasonable downtime between sessions.

5

SOME RECOMMENDED COMPONENTS

This book isn't about finding your lady to serve or finding your devoted servant. We think the question of finding others in the BDSM community is a widely covered topic and we don't need to recover old material beyond a few words. If you want to find someone you have to go where the people interested in BDSM are going. Workshops, munches, lectures, readings, conventions: become part of the action and you will both see and be seen.

If you want to find someone you can build an owner-slave or 24/7 relationship with, you will need a lot of time to find a compatible person, evaluate each other, try things out, and then work on creating a connection that goes beyond the bedroom or dungeon.

This section of our book is about how you can use contracts, rituals, rules, protocols, and training to help you set up your dynamic so you can nurture it into a stable, serious, and long-term relationship. We will not claim that our views of these five topics are the Gospel of Kink, but we've used them and continue to use them, and we've seen them used in almost every single long-term M/s couple and household we respect.

CONTRACTS

Creating and using contracts may be one of the most hotly debated topics in the BDSM community, especially online where people claim right and left that they never had one and will never use one, along with pooh-poohing the idea of safewords. Within dynamics, contracts can also create tension, as we ourselves have seen, when the value of said contracts is different for each person.

An M/s contract is usually a written document where both people in a relationship agree about the parameters of their relationship. Let us be perfectly clear: we have never, ever known a BDSM or M/s contract to have any legal standing in any part of the Western world. Some couples do consult legal counsel after years together to set up appropriate paperwork to grant rights similar to marriage, while others simply get married to provide some legal protections for both parties. The contract we are talking about in this book has no legal authority.

It has a much higher authority: Honor. The contract's value is only as good as the honesty and integrity of the parties who design it and sign it. As soon as one of you decides, consciously or unconsciously, that the terms listed in that contract no longer matter, the contract and the relationship it created are well on the way to an end — if not outright destroyed.

Some people don't like contracts. Over the years, Fox grew to deeply dislike our contract, which developed from a very detailed training contract TammyJo created over several years (which you can read in the Appendix) into a renewed slave owning contract that basically made a few adjustments for changes in our life. This proved to be quite a disagreement between us, and it almost broke us up, because for TammyJo, the idea of a contract was almost akin to a marriage license, though frankly more useful in her opinion. For Fox, the idea that he needed his relationship spelled out seemed artificial, and after about three years together, he wanted it all to feel "natural." He wanted to provide good service and be obedient since this is how the relationship worked not because he was following a list. The result was a very short three-paragraph contract that has been our contract since the spring of 2002. It says:

Fox loves TammyJo.

And for that love, he promises to do what he can to assure his Mistress, TammyJo, that he does.

He promises to console her when she is sad and celebrate with her when she is happy.

TammyJo promises not to harm her slave, Fox, intentionally — to show concern for his mental, physical, and emotional welfare.

This contract shall serve until such time as a more formal contract is devised.

Dated and signed by both parties.

We cannot recommend that anyone have a contract like ours to begin a relationship. Look at it. It is very vague, and indeed it has been interpreted as merely a continuation of the much longer contracts by TammyJo and thus has been accepted by Fox to mean the same thing. There's no "out" here, since he agreed to "do what he can." In turn she really gained a lot of authority and power in this contract, because "harm" can be vague, though you've seen our beliefs on that, and "concern" is amazingly vague and can be either active or passive. If we were super picky about words, this tiny contract would not have lasted the eight years it has. Instead we realize that we have to work together to make our dynamic function well for both of us.

For those of you starting out, though, having more details can lessen your arguments and help the dominant get a deeper understanding of where her authority lies and the limitations she should keep in mind when exercising it. For the submissive, having this reference can help you review and practice what is important. Practice? Oh, yeah, there will be practice for both of you, which we'll get to in the Training section of this chapter. You'll find a copy of our last, long, detailed contract in the appendix.

Ultimately any contract, legal or private, has the value you both place on it, so don't just copy someone else's and stick your names into it. Definitely look around at books, talk to others, and even consult online for examples of contracts, but don't copy them without a good deal of thought. TammyJo did research for an entire year before designing her training contract and then revised it over the next few years to reflect reality. What do they have in common? There are several good books TammyJo consulted that you might want to read for advice about what to include in a contract.[1] Please consult the latest editions of any of these books, because they will have updated medical and legal advice. How can you incorporate your needs and wants into the contract? What will realistically work for you day in and day out? We'll address some specifics in the section on rules, rituals and protocols that you might want to put into a contract.

---

[1] Larry Townsend, *The Leatherman's Handbook II* (New York: Carlyle Communications, inc., 1985); John Warren, Ph.D., *The (new and improved) Loving Dominant* (Eugene, OR: Greenery Press, 2009); Pat Califia, *Sensuous Magic: A Guide to S/M for Adventurous Couples* (San Francisco: Cleis Press, 2002); Race Bannon, *Learning the Ropes: A Basic Guide to Safe and Fun S/M Lovemaking* (Los Angeles: Daedalus Publishing Company, 1992); Dossie Easton and Janet W. Hardy, *The New Bottoming Book* (Oakland, CA: Greenery Press, 2001); Dossie Easton and Janet W. Hardy, *The New Topping Book* (Oakland, CA: Greenery Press, 2003). We have left out self-published books.

If one of you has more experience, especially if that person is the dominant, feel free to write out a standard contract you can show to your partner. Just remember that you may need to modify it for your particular situation and health over time, because situations are going to change as you get older and as economic conditions shift. As you each get more experience, either with each other or with other people, you will learn things about yourself that may necessitate changing a standard contract as well. Don't reject a sample contract from an experienced submissive, because it is not uncommon for the submissive partner to have more experience, especially if a vanilla relationship between you two existed before any D/s or M/s came into the picture.

If you are that more experienced submissive and you want to design a contract, think long and hard about fantasy vs. reality when you do so. It is very easy to think you can handle a lot of supervision by your dominant; in fact, it may be a big turn-on for you. But day after day, week after week, everything you agree to needs to flow and be easily maintained until it feels natural to you. The more specifics you put into your contract, the less room you give your owner to grow and exercise her authority, the one thing your relationship is built around. The more detailed the rituals, rules and protocols, the less easily you'll be able to demonstrate your loyalty and devotion in ways designed to make her life easier and allow your submission to shine.

Fox has a very strong piece of advice: ***Don't sign anything you can't support.***

This is a matter of your personal honor, so if you think you may have difficulty keeping up a list of fifty things the slave or the owner must do, don't sign it. Work on making a contract that will be acceptable to you both. If you can't find that, then you may not be compatible. There is no shame in realizing it won't work or isn't working, but a good deal of harm might be done if you continue to build up resentments over rules and duties you just can't do on a regular basis.

Rituals, Rules, & Protocols

In this section we are going to address three interrelated systems that are commonly used and abused, and often argued about, within the BDSM community. These are rituals, rules and protocols that can be used to help strengthen your M/s dynamic, but can also lead to serious problems unless you choose wisely which to use every day, for private scenes and for public occasions.

Contrary to what many online would have you believe, there has never been a set of guidelines for any of these things. Claims of using "Old Guard" or "European House" systems do not reflect historical evidence. "Old Guard" is a modern term created to describe the codes of the various gay biker clubs that existed in the USA after WWII. Although there were commonalities between these groups, there was no universal code. Unless you are a WWII vet yourself and a gay man, it's unlikely you were "Old Guard," though you may have learned from these forefathers. As for "European Houses," there is frankly no evidence for them beyond whispers or online bragging. If such places really existed, they must have operated in secret and were the privilege of the elites in each area, and their practices probably ran counter to the laws and mores of the greater societies in which they supposedly existed. Their rituals, rules and protocols are therefore unlikely to have been handed down to just anyone, assuming they were real in the first place, because that would run the risk of spreading their secrets. The fact is that before the second half of the 20th century there was nothing that we would today consider an organized BDSM community and therefore no set of "true" or "traditional" rules.

Guess what? It doesn't matter anyway, because unless you join an organization or attend a party with its own rituals, rules and protocols in place, you only need to worry about what will help your relationship stay grounded on an M/s foundation. Your rules can be incorporated into your contract, or they can be developed over time. While most of these systems are imposed by the dominant, some of them can also be created by or insisted upon by the submissive. We'll talk about each category and the benefits and problems you can expect with each; we'll also try to simplify the definitions and give examples for each type of system you can use in your relationship. This is a huge topic that has been covered in the books we've previously footnoted as well as a couple of newer books[2]. Since we don't want you to just copy our rituals, rules and protocols, we may be a bit vague at times about the particular words we use.

Think of rituals as those actions and words you use repeatedly to help create a certain emotional and mental environment. These can be things you do yourself or with your partner. For example, a slave who gets up every morning, looks in the mirror, and says out loud, "Today I will honor myself and my mistress by being the best I can be," is performing a ritual that helps ground him for the day ahead. The lady who takes a bath and then puts on a certain pair of

---

2   Robert J. Rubel, PhD, *Protocol Handbook for the Leather Slave: Theory and Practice* (Las Vegas: The Nazca Plains Corporation, 2006); Machele Kindle, *Manual Creation: Defining the Structure of an M/s Household* (Las Vegas: The Nazca Plains Corporation, 2006); Robert J. Rubel, PhD, *Protocols: A Variety of Views* (Las Vegas: The Nazca Plains Corporation, 2008). We have left out self-published books.

boots before picking up her crop and starting a scene is also performing a ritual to help ground her for the activities she is about to direct. Rituals can therefore be used daily or for special occasions, but their main purpose is to help you get into a certain mindset.

In our household we have a few rituals that might help you see what is possible. Instead of a traditional collar, Fox had his ears pierced to mark our seventh anniversary. However, since the collar is a widely respected symbol in the BDSM community, we use his whenever we go to a public event. This is how our ritual goes: TammyJo gets the collar or asks Fox to fetch it. She holds it open in her hands while he kneels down. We look into each others' eyes, and then, as she places it around his neck, she states what this represents and why he is allowed to wear it and asks him what it represents for him. He answers and then kneels into what we call "First Position" until she taps one foot. This reminds us both that out in public we represent the household within the greater community and mentally preps us for stepping out, especially if it's a special event or among strangers. To be blunt, since TammyJo has a bit of a name in the greater community, it is important that we never forget to be on our best behavior in public.

We have an evening ritual that we use every day just to ground ourselves with the knowledge that no matter what the rest of the day has been like, here we are, two people who support and love each other in what could be considered an unusual fashion that works well for us. At bedtime, Fox removes TammyJo's shoes and socks and kisses each of her feet, then we hug and are silent (or at least try to be) for a few moments, just being with each other. These few moments of reassurance are so important that when we must miss an evening due to travel we both feel a great sense of loss. Even when one of us is ill, the other makes sure to accommodate the other's need to participate in this ritual so we can complete our day as a couple.

Rituals work best if they are geared toward the individual and the couple; this is simply because they have to affect your state of mind and no one else's. What works for you one year may not work the next because of other matters in your life. TammyJo used to ritually sort through all of her equipment, drawers and racks of it, before a scene, but now she just gets the tools she needs and lays them out in an orderly fashion. As she's gained more confidence she no longer feels the need to go through every single one and set it up properly. These are rituals because, beyond mental and emotional grounding, they do not dictate what we do or how we do things. Rules and protocols take things a bit further.

Rules set the limits of what you each can and can't do. Often they are assumed to be limitations and directions for the slave or submissive to follow, but let us be clear. Unless the owner knows these rules inside and out, and unless she is willing to enforce them consistently, the rules mean nothing and in fact may harm your relationship. TammyJo can testify to this firsthand. She once had a slave who wanted a lot of rules and protocols. She was rather neutral about them, but since this seemed so important to him, she agreed, and they set up some fairly elaborate rules about his seeing her every day and at certain times, communicating every night. There were other rules about how he was to do various things she can't even remember. Being a woman of her word, she enforced these. In the end he tossed those rules back at her, claiming she was abusing him by making him follow them, and she learned a good lesson: Never agree to rules as the dominant if you are not behind them 100%.

We never claimed any of this was equal or fair in the vanilla sense. As a slave you may very well be presented with rules that you feel neutral about, and you may be required to follow them or end the relationship. Your role here is to obey, not to enforce, so your passion for the rules is less necessary to the stability of the dynamic. A good example of this is our rule about TammyJo's name never being used in private as anything other than a safeword. This rule was important to her because one of the ways she trained herself to be safe and consensual was to have a mundane signal that she would recognize immediately as a signal that there was a problem. Since titles turn her on and are unique to the D/s or M/s dynamic, being called by her title is very important to her. It is a non-negotiable rule. To be blunt, sometimes Fox just isn't feeling the passion behind saying "Mistress" to her, yet he tries very hard to follow this rule because he has seen the dramatic difference in her attitude and behavior when he calls her TammyJo.

Even as a slave, though, you should never agree to a rule you hate, because you will develop resentment. If you discover over time that you do indeed hate a rule, then bring that up and see if it can be negotiated. Depending on why the rule is in effect, it may be changed or eliminated, but don't be surprised if a rule has strong meaning to the dominant and becomes a deal-breaker. Better to get out than to continue poisoning the relationship by trying to follow a rule that makes you feel horrible.

One example of modified rules concerns the "Slave Positions" (which you'll read about in just a moment). Because of a physical issue with Fox's knees and ankles, he is unable to kneel for extended periods without his legs going numb. When Fox realized this was going to be a problem with satisfying Mistress' standard design, he asked if position #6 could be modified. Acknowledging that modifying the position was in our best interest (given that the whole point of the positions was to create a focused mindset), she worked with Fox to modify the position to something he could sustain. Now, Fox could have remained silent, trapped in the viewpoint that a good slave would just grin and bear it, but the resulting effects (namely, the pain and numbness) would eventually have prevented him from being able to follow Mistress' directions, or at the very least would have distracted him from focusing on her.

The definition of protocols can overlap with that of rules, but we think what sets these two categories apart is scope and purpose. Rules establish limits, while protocols are guides to how you should behave and are often part of a couple or household's public performance of their dynamic. Both rules and protocols can be listed and written in the contract, but we believe that rules must be clearly stated, while protocols can develop more organically — though then they need to be clarified so that everyone knows how to behave. We know, that's as clear as mud, so let's give you some examples from what we readily admit is our low-protocol household.

Protocols are guidelines for how you should behave. There are protocols for slaves, yes, but also for owners, as well as between people of the same and different ranks, and these also vary by situation. We are a low-protocol household, but we do have some protocols that also fit under the "Rules" category.

One such protocol that we have is the set of "Slave Positions" that are taught and practiced during the "Training Phase" of a relationship then used with varying degrees of frequency when we move into ownership. The meaning of the positions is to help each of us to get into a particular state of mind. For the dominant, seeing a position adopted by your submissive is simply arousing, because it displays your authority and often presents the submissive's body in an attractive fashion. For the submissive, it serves to focus your attention and prepare yourself mentally for the function related to the given stance (inspection, presenting an item, presenting oneself for punishment, etc). It also serves as a non-verbal form of communication, allowing the submissive to indicate a need or desire without having to ask for it vocally — which can be hard for some people. Fox is well aware that TammyJo might say "Position seven" or "Three" at any time, so he practices the positions privately, both to show his commitment to the dynamic and his respect for her protocols and because it's embarrassing not to know how to perform on command.

Since many "slave positions" are based on female submissives, TammyJo modified and adapted them for men. If you are the dominant, try that. Don't necessarily copy; modify to fit what you like and want — this includes the ones in the sample training contract you'll find in the appendices to this book. Have some flexibility built into them for physical limitations that will change from person to person and over time. If you are the submissive, it is fine to find a set of positions you like and practice them, but remember that if you insist on using only yours, you are undermining the authority of your potential dominant right from the start, and that is not a very good foundation to build upon.

Other protocols we follow relate to how we interact with other people in a BDSM or leather setting. First, if the meeting or event has its own rules, we follow those. To do otherwise is disrespectful, and it is better to stay away from an organization whose protocols rub you the wrong way than it is to upset everyone by refusing to follow them. Second, we both try to practice simple etiquette. For Fox this means saying "Sir" or "Ma'am" to unknown tops, and for both of us it means first getting permission from a top before speaking to their submissive. It also means never, ever touching anyone or anything that is not ours without an invitation. TammyJo gets a lot of compliments on how polite Fox is, and she honestly just can't take too much credit for that, because his parents raised him to be a gentleman. Remember, build off the strengths your partner already has and your foundation will be much stronger.

We don't care how often you see "femdoms" running around in porn or even at events touching everything and everyone and demanding they be called "Lady" or "Mistress" or whatever. Such behavior is rude and gives all female dominants a bad reputation. Likewise, regardless of how many male submissives you see bowing and scraping and begging, doing that feeds the idea that men are only interested in themselves and their fetishes. Please remember that when you go out in public, even if it is a private kink event, you are representing not just yourself but the entire community and anyone with the same orientation. You wouldn't want us to show you in a bad light, so be polite and respectful until you get permission to be otherwise.

Those who misbehave in these ways have no protocols or just plain bad protocols — probably drawn from porn or fantasies. You can be low- or high-protocol and still function quite well in private and in public. There are many discussions and even some books about protocols that you can consult. Again, never copy these as-is into your life, but do try them out during the training phase and see what works best at supporting your relationship every day and in special situations.

By this point you're probably wondering why we don't have a chapter or a section about punishments. The answer is easy: Punishments vary greatly in their form, their use and their purpose. To thoroughly discuss the multitude of questions that have been raised online, at munches, in groups, in books, between partners, and within households would require far more time than we want to give it. But we will briefly address this issue here.

First, punishment is not an excuse for SM or play time. You can call that "funishment"[3] if you like, but to confuse it with actual punishment, meaning correction that is meant to bring about a change in behavior, is to truly confuse your dynamic, as well as your partner and yourself. Punishment is not meant to be fun for either partner, because it represents a failure in your dynamic, either on the part of the Mistress, who may not have trained well or communicated clearly, or on the part of the slave, who may have chosen to disobey or to act contrary to the desired nature of the relationship. We don't know about you, but failure of any type hurts us deeply, and we do everything in our power to avoid it.

Second, you need to decide early on whether punishment is going to be part of your dynamic. If it is, then you need to be very clear about what actions or attitudes will result in punishment. "Funishment" is great for the short term or an isolated scene, but we're talking about creating a lifetime together, and you need stable ground to build upon. In our relationship, punishment is only given for willful disobedience. We can still count on one hand after eleven years the number of times that Fox has been formally punished. That isn't to say he's perfect or that TammyJo is perfect, but willful disobedience is quite different from making errors or mistakes, which are just part of being human. There are always consequences for your actions, both of your actions, but those consequences may not be punishments in the formal sense.

Finally, we really want to caution you about doing anything as a punishment that you would enjoy in another context. The fact is that human beings learn to associate behaviors and actions very strongly; what might be a fun spanking or an arousing spanking can turn sour if it's also how you punish. The long-term couples and households we know of who use punishment do something that is different from their SM or bondage play. Punishment also will vary from slave to slave and from situation to situation.

Changing behavior and upholding your relationship should be the purpose of punishment. If the same actions or attitudes keep coming up repeatedly, you need to seriously re-evaluate your methods and reasons. Re-evaluation does not make you a weak owner; it makes you a smart one. Likewise, repeating offenses

---

3   A term that arose on the Internet many years ago, although who created it first is unclear.

doesn't make you a SAM (Smart-Ass Masochist); it simply makes you annoying and perhaps unworthy of her time.

Remember, the rules, rituals, and protocols only work to maintain your relationship if you both support them, use them, and make sure they become part of your daily life. Anything short of that will undermine the foundations you are trying to build upon. We'll discuss how to maintain that foundation in a positive and powerful fashion in the next chapter.

Training

Think of training as receiving or giving knowledge that will help you fulfill a role, perform a task, or lay the groundwork for further education. An experience requires at least three things to be considered training by our standards. First, a controlled situation where an activity or sensation is explored. Second, feedback on how things went and possible corrections or changes. Third, opportunities to practice, practice, practice, with a focus on improvement.

Normally we think of training in BDSM as something the dominant does to the submissive. That way of thinking seriously undermines the value of training for dominants and obscures the reality of how it functions. This is why we're going to tackle the training of owners before moving on to slave training.

Dominants are often hesitant to say they are "trained," perhaps because it sounds like they have been in a lower position. Well, you have been. There was a time when you didn't know what you know now, and there are things you still don't know how to do. It is a simple fact that every single dominant out there had to learn in some way. Even if it was by trial and error, they were learning, and learning is part of training. When you look up information and practice it on your own, you are still training yourself – and, hopefully, giving yourself room to make mistakes, admit them, and keep practicing until you feel confident.

Dominants can also be trained by others. You can attend workshops or lectures hosted by kinky groups or as part of a convention. You can seek out other dominants to mentor you, which means they share their experiences with you, often teaching you specific techniques. TammyJo learned to do flogging, bondage, and knife play while in New York City from tops she got to know and respected. She calls that time of her life her apprenticeship in BDSM. A mentor should be a guide, helping you learn by asking questions, offering examples and correcting your errors in terms of physical play. They are not a god, nor are they the only model around which you should construct your identity or style as a dominant. In fact, TammyJo strongly suggests you get as much variety as you can in terms of learning from other dominants. Since you are a woman, obviously another female dominant might have experience you could benefit from. But a gay or even het male top can also have a lot to offer you. Limiting yourself to only people of the same orientation, both in terms of sexuality and BDSM, is limiting your ability to gain as much knowledge and experience as you can.

As a dominant, and as an owner, very few things are more sexy and inspiring to submissives and slaves than knowledge and experience. That creates a catch-22. Without time and information, without the ability to act like you know what you are doing and to talk like you have more than just a clue, most submissives won't give you the time of day unless they are really just interested in sex, a topic we'll cover later in this book. Submissives want someone to whom they can entrust their bodies, hearts, minds, and sometimes souls, and they'd be fools to just randomly turn that power and authority over to anyone. Slaves want someone worthy of their devotion and daily service, and that's difficult to give if their owner doesn't really know what she needs or wants. So in terms of finding a lifetime slave, you need to get all the training or education you can get. Plus it will make you feel more confident, which cranks up your dominance.

In many circles there is a knee-jerk reaction to the idea that a submissive might be able to train a dominant. Fine. Call it something else if it makes you feel better, but the fact remains that you are learning about things and expanding your repertoire of activities and styles you can incorporate into your life. TammyJo learned something with each person she trained, each dominant she spoke to, and from each workshop or lecture she attended and continues to attend. Learning from submissives helped her fine-tune her empathy and gave her other perspectives to draw from, both for her play and in her writing. At the very least you must be open to listening to any submissive you play with and paying attention to any slave you own in order to do things safely and consensually. Learning from them then becomes a natural bonus.

Dominants can also bottom or submit as part of their becoming more confident dominants and more skilled tops. The "bottom route" was actually a big part of many Old Guard groups and became a mantra for the online and print "New Guard" community back in the 1990s. This approach can be tricky for several reasons.

First, if you don't feel you will honestly benefit from bottoming, it won't do you any good. Just like going to a class and sitting there but never taking notes, never doing the homework, and never really thinking about the material won't help you pass a college class, just showing up and going through the motions isn't going to help you much. It might not be just a matter of what you feel either. TammyJo tried the "bottom route" herself and discovered her personality made it almost impossible for any dominant or top to feel they were really connecting; some ended things because of the unconsciously negative vibes she gave off.

Secondly, each human being processes sensation differently, and each of us has a unique background that filters what we experience. Thus no two people will feel a whip the same way or respond to a command with identical emotional reactions. This is a fact that you have to be able to fully grasp if bottoming is going to help you learn anything about being a dominant.

Sadly we've met some people over the years who did the "bottom route" first, and who developed a very negative attitude about bottoms and subs. They assume that anything they could handle could be done by anyone. They are unable to empathize, or to understand that others will perceive pain and pleasure differently from them. They constantly compare their own experiences and feelings on the bottom side to what they believe their partners should be doing. This isn't a problem of bottoming, though, but of a general lack of empathy coupled with an inflated ego. For some people, "the bottom route" helped them, and if you think it will help you, then go for it, but be honest with your top or dominant that you believe this is a step to your own identity as a Mistress in the future. Doing so might help lessen hurt feelings when the time comes for you to move into that other role or to add it to your life.

A third problem with the bottom route for dominants is how you may be perceived by others. In general we haven't found a distrust or a dislike from other dominants; indeed, among some organizations starting on the bottom is part of how their community functions. We have seen and heard a lot of negative comments from submissives about dominants who bottomed in the past and even more negative reactions to those who decide they are switches and wish to keep submission or bottoming in their lives. Some people strongly feel they could never kneel to someone who has ever been on the other side or that they'd always worry they might lose their dominant to a more "masterly" top.

That's a depressing reality for those who choose this way to learn, and for switches. There is good news: Not everyone feels this way. If a potential partner responds negatively to the fact you trained as a submissive first or that you enjoy bottoming, we suggest just moving on to the next possible relationship. Submissives aren't that rare; there are many you can find if you keep your eyes open and are honest about what you need and want.

The commonest and best understood form of training is, of course, a dominant training a submissive. Usually this is their own submissive, but training can be done more objectively by another person; TammyJo has done this for a few couples in the past and for individuals who wanted a safe person to learn from before they made any sort of personal commitment. An example of her standard training contract can be found in the Appendix.

A lot of dubious activities can be called "training" by people, especially in pornography. We apply the same definition of training here as we did for the top role. Training a slave means giving knowledge that will help the slave fulfill a role, perform a task, or lay the groundwork for further education. In this case the slave is learning how to serve, how different sensations feel, and how to understand his reactions to being obedient to another. Simply getting fucked is not being trained, simply being flogged is not being trained, and simply being yelled at for dropping a plate is not being trained.

If you are a would-be slave, you can train yourself. It will be more difficult, though, because without a top or dominant a lot of it will be merely theory, and reality can be quite different. Eventually you must get out of your head and entrust someone to help you understand what that flogger feels like, at the very least. If you want to explore on your own, any of the books we've noted in the footnotes are great ways to begin exploring. We don't believe that books should be off-limits to anyone simply based on their orientation. However, there are some books specifically designed to help would-be slaves figure things out a bit better, and we can recommend a few[4]. Never consider your solo training to be the end of learning to serve,. The fact is that most owners want things done in unique ways and like to take some time to teach you to do things their way. Getting too set in what you believe is the best way to do something is going to prove a hurdle to a new relationship, whether you learned those "ways" on your own or in earlier dynamics.

Those same books can be used by would-be owners as well to design a training program. We are perhaps a bit old-fashioned and a bit too academic, but a purposeful program will result in more easily-learned rules, rituals, and protocols as well as offer positive opportunities for improvement without the confusion that can happen from random moments of training. When TammyJo

---

[4] A grateful slave with guy Baldwin, M.S., *SlaveCraft, Roadmaps for Erotic Servitude: principles, skills and tools* (Los Angeles: Daedalus Publishing company, 2002); Jack Rinella, *Becoming a Slave: The Theory & Practice of Voluntary Servitude* (Chicago: Rinella Editorial services, 2005). We have left out self-published books.

refined her training contract she had access to two new books that are now published as one.[5] Fox and others she trained after this point were required to read these books and complete the exercises in them, along with exercises TammyJo created. For her, as a college professor, this was a very familiar and useful method to help her and the submissive determine whether they were a good match and whether slavery was really what that submissive honestly wanted. For Fox, the training allowed him to qualify and quantify those aspects of submission that he enjoyed and those that he had no interest in whatsoever. It also clarified that while he would be able to sustain a D/s relationship with TammyJo, it was not something he was looking for with anyone else. Fox is not just anyone's slave. He is TammyJo's slave. Understanding that distinction is very important before you begin any BDSM relationship.

The key to successful training for both the owner and the slave is a commitment to take the process seriously. If you have homework assignments, you need to do them. If are you asked to express your thoughts, you must struggle to comply as honestly as you can. If you have a schedule for training, a day of the week you meet, or a particular time of day, you must both be on time and be prepared for the activities you are about to undertake. If the tasks or assignments seem boring, that might simply reflect that this particular way of doing things isn't the best for you. Bring this issue up with your partner, regardless of your role. Training won't provide the solid foundation for your relationship unless you can both use it to help create an M/s dynamic that is going to function day in and day out.

Training is when you try out those rules, those rituals, and those protocols. The point is for those you decide to keep and incorporate into your owner-slave relationship to become second nature to you by the time training is done. You may have heard the expression that training is never done. Frankly, we think that's misusing the concept of training. If a submissive isn't 90% trained by the time you decide to move on to owning him, perhaps you didn't do it correctly. Ownership should be a time of use and pleasure in one's property, not merely a continuation of the pre-M/s dynamic under different titles. For slaves, being owned should be about being allowed to serve in the best ways you can, not worrying about being constantly corrected or having new methods of doing things created over and over.

---

5   Christina Abernathy, *Miss Abernathy's Concise Slave Training Manual* (San Francisco: Greenery Press, 1996); Christina Abernathy, *Training with Miss Abernathy: a workbook for erotic slaves and their owners* (San Francisco: Greenery Press, 1998). Now published as a single volume as *Erotic Slavehood* (Oakland, CA: Greenery Press, 2007).

Keeping a slave off balance is something a lot of dominants like to do, or so they say, but in reality most people function best with consistent rules, rituals, protocols and expectations. As an owner, your life will be much happier when your slave's service is smooth, efficient and motivated by the desire to please, not merely the fear of punishment. Not to mention how much more free time you as the owner will have in your life with a well-trained slave you don't have to repeatedly correct or instruct. Note that we didn't say training is 100% finished, because life changes, and what works one week or one year may not work the next.

Yes, this does mean that training is going to take some time. TammyJo's formal introductory training program was a 14-week program where she met for 3-5 hours once a week with a potential slave and assigned about that same amount of homework each week. As the trainer she had to keep up on all that work herself and stay on top of it, so it also required effort, time and energy from her. This is why she has never trained for fun, only for a partner with strong potential or on behalf of a couple she respected and felt might benefit. She expected the same effort, time and energy from the trainee, and she could quickly tell when someone couldn't or didn't take the process seriously enough for her. They'd show up without homework done, or they'd put off taking a community class that cost $15 for a semester's worth of sessions. Or they'd just answer too quickly to be letting the activities and protocols they were practicing really affect them.

Why should you invest this much time? Remember what we talked about in terms of getting to know a person before you jump into a scene with them or into a relationship? We saw training as a middle ground between that "getting to know you" stage and ownership. When you try out the rules you think you want to use every day, you learn over the course of weeks whether or not it will be feasible. A person can pretend for a session or two or maybe a week or two, but repeatedly doing something either becomes second nature or a huge annoyance. Also, trainees can easily investigate their fantasies over these weeks and repeated practice sessions. In fantasy it might be very sexy to be kept naked, but you might discover in reality that you get uncomfortable after a while and that the chill distracts you from performing to the best of your ability. Having someone at your beck and call, just waiting in the corner of the room, might be hot to think about, but you might discover that you feel limited in your daily actions by such a constant presence. Isn't it better to discover these differences between your fantasies now rather than once you've signed a contract, made a verbal commitment, or worse yet moved in together?

Let's use ourselves and our past experiences to demonstrate. TammyJo "owned" a boy for about a month or two after some playing around together and talking at a local BDSM organization. She owned Faith for 18 months after putting him through her very serious 14-week training period. She's owned Fox for more than a decade after almost 30 weeks of serious training. It really helped us learn about each other when we took the time to train with a purpose before jumping into the next level of D/s. M/s isn't innately better than D/s, but it is different, and we urge you to take it slowly and purposefully so you increase your chances for long-term success.

6

FOUNDATIONS OF OWNER/SLAVE DYNAMICS

What makes a Mistress-slave relationship work in the long term? You can get to know each other slowly, do some serious training, and have everything grounded in reality, and it can still fail. We want to talk about eight different subjects that we believe have helped us last this long and this intensely, compared to our previous relationships where the people involved proved to be mismatched in terms of one or more of these categories. If a lot of this sounds vanilla at first, if these sound like very mundane issues that any couple can have, you're right; it is, and they are. At its core, M/s is in reality a human relationship where the authority difference has been mutually recognized and is supported by everyone involved. That is the biggest and most important difference between owning someone or being owned, and living together or being married.

Commitment

Obviously in order for the authority structure to work, you both have to be committed to supporting it. Anyone can say the words, "I want to do this," or, "I believe in us." A lot of people seem to have little trouble signing documents without much thought. Tons of folks are running around online and offline spouting all sorts of romantic BS about erotic slavery and then having fits when their partner's initially intense interest changes or decreases. It is easy to say the words, but commitment is more about actions than mere words.

A person who agrees to a set of rules, rituals and protocols and then needs to be constantly reminded of them demonstrates that they are not committed to the dynamic. If they were, those behaviors would flow from them. Oh, not right away; that's what the training period was partly for, but if months of ownership have passed, or even years, and you still find yourself unable to remember to bow when entering your owner's room or forgetting to call her by her preferred title, then you need to stop and assess what is going on inside of you that is making you resist what is supposed to be a consensual arrangement.

A similar thing can happen to a self-proclaimed owner. You stop enforcing your contract's details, you stop telling your partner to do the things you agreed you'd control, or you get angry at the idea of making yet another decision. You just start floating around expecting things to get done without exercising your authority or taking the responsibilities you promised you would. If that happens, you have to stop and try to figure out what has changed in your life.

There are constant challenges to your commitment to maintain this authority dynamic. We'll talk about many of these in the next chapter, but just to foreshadow them now, these challenges can range from economic conditions to family obligations to just plain losing that spark that made you want to get into this relationship to begin with. It is when these challenges happen that the test of your commitment begins.

Who can make you obey? You the slave make that decision. The owner might punish you, but obedience — honest, sincere obedience — comes from an internal desire to please and a need for direction.

Who can make you, the owner, step up and exercise your authority? You make that decision. Your slave can tell you he needs more from you, but short of walking out that door and ending it all, he can't force you to do something with your full heart and mind behind it.

Ignoring rough periods and acting like nothing is wrong is a set-up for resentments to build over time. Commitment to the relationship also includes being honest about problems and being willing to make the effort necessary to assess them and then overcome them. If you find you just feel physically too tired to do chores or enforce rules, then you need to take care of your health so you are less tired. If you find you feel annoyed by giving orders or obeying, then you need to try to determine when your feelings changed.

Daily rituals can be a great way to help you enforce your commitment to each other. Think of it as a time to reconnect with each other in a formal way that emphasizes your authority differences. This is partly what we do every night when Fox kneels to remove TammyJo's shoes. Rules must be enforced, or they have no more value; thus, TammyJo won't respond to hearing her first name from Fox (assuming he isn't having serious problems that require discussion), which reinforces the fact that she has a title that he is to use. Protocols also need to be enforced, so before taking overtime at work or joining a gathering with his friends, Fox checks in to make sure he can be free at that time, submitting to TammyJo's decision should it be "No."

Another approach to improving your commitment is just to make yourself do something and smile while you do it. The idea here is that by doing and acting like you are happy, you can convince yourself that you want to do this and whatever "this" is becomes second nature. Frankly, we think this strategy only works if there is strong underlying commitment to the dynamic already. If you've lost interest in your partner or in M/s or D/s, that happens because people change over time. By then, no amount of pretending is going to make it feel good or normal to you. Try "acting as if" early, when you first find yourself lagging in your commitment to the relationship, before bad habits become ingrained.

Finally, never forget to communicate when you hit a rough patch. Being committed isn't just words, but it isn't just actions either. Words and actions have to match, so use your words and pay attention to your dominant's or submissive's attitude and behavior. Many relationships end before the people involved discover that they had problems they might have been able to solve if they'd only had the courage to talk about them and work on things together.

That's the real key. You are in a relationship with another person, and possibly more than one if you are polyamorous. You can't do it yourself. You can carry on as though nothing is wrong, fooling yourself for a while, but eventually you'll get frustrated enough that you bitch about things online or at a local munch or in a vanilla situation. That frustration will turn to resentment and anger if you realize your partner isn't putting in the work (or, in other words, isn't as committed to your dynamic as you are). When those negative emotions start showing up, the lifespan of your M/s dynamic is starting to tick down.

Remember, commitment to your relationship is also a commitment to yourself — a promise that you will do what you need to do in order to live the life you want. You desire the best, so give your relationship your best effort.

Loyalty

One way commitment is challenged is through opportunities to be disloyal to your partner, yourself, and the relationship. When we put a formal slave collar on

Fox before public events where we know that symbol will have more value than those we use daily, Fox and I exchange a few sentences that are a ritual we use to help ground us before venturing out into the kinky world. Part of the ritual is a proclamation of loyalty on Fox's behalf. It wasn't something that TammyJo thought of, but it is something that is very important to him.

There are several different things that require your loyalty in order to make your relationship work long-term. First, you need to be loyal to yourself, not betray your own morals and ethics, stick up for yourself, and not allow yourself to be harmed if you can in any way prevent that. Let's be honest: if you aren't all there, if you aren't giving your best and being at your best, you can hardly give your best to another person. This might mean you do some rather unsubmissive things at times to protect yourself, or it might be that you stop yourself from overextending yourself in the name of some almighty dominance you want to portray to the world. In other words, loyalty to yourself is respecting yourself.

You also have to be loyal to the person you've made a commitment to be in this relationship with. In a way this is a matter of semantics, because in order to keep your commitment you need to be loyal in the first place — or do you? Let's say that you promised to obey your dominant but your dominant has never mentioned that you might need to defend her honor in public. Then at a munch when she goes to the restroom someone makes a snippy comment about her that you know to be incorrect. You might think that as a submissive the most you can do is tell her about it later, but being loyal means standing up for her at that moment, because silence is the same as agreement in such a situation. The exact same situation might arise but with the roles reversed, though usually people are more cautious about badmouthing a slave around his owner.

Commitment is the work you put into the relationship and honoring the promises you made. Loyalty is going beyond that and defending your relationship whenever and under whatever circumstances arise. That can be scary. What if your boss at work found out you keep a slave at home? Are you brave enough to point out that your private life is just that, private, or will you be disloyal to your dynamic and try to make excuses or, worse yet, deny it? You might think you have no choice, but your heart knows that by denying your relationship, you've shown you aren't loyal to it.

Loyalty and commitment aren't switches you turn on or off when it's convenient or when it's easy. They must be a fundamental part of your relationship that both of you exercise. That isn't true for all of the foundational blocks of your M/s dynamic. Some of the categories we are discussing seem more appropriate for one role than the other – until you look very closely at how they work in reality.

SELFISHNESS

Selfishness is mostly a dominant quality that owners need to work on to make a successful M/s dynamic last for years and years. While the bulk of this section is going to be focused on the ladies, we want to say a few words first about how selfishness can be important for slaves to have, as well as a potential killer to a relationship.

There are two main areas where selfishness is a good thing for a slave. The first is protection. At the end of the day, at the end of life, the only person you can ever say truly had the ability to protect you is you. Being able to express your limits is a good thing; it is selfishness in a positive sense. Contrary to what online "experts" say, every one of us has limits, because we're all just human beings. Giving your potential owner information about your limits is necessary and remains important throughout your relationship, because people change over time. However, selfishness in this sense goes a step further. If you are involved with someone who won't respect your limits, you need to respect yourself enough to walk away. This isn't topping from the bottom at all. This is protecting the property that you are – if not for this unworthy person who isn't respecting you, then for the woman who will someday be a good match as your Mistress.

Don't confuse using selfishness to protect yourself with undermining your owner's authority. Undermining happens when a slave claims that something is a limit, simply because he's decided he doesn't like to do it or that it is a challenge to him. Here's the problem: A good owner can't read your mind, they can't see if you are lying or not, and they have to trust you when you say something has become a limit for you. You can get away with controlling the relationship via false limits, but eventually you will be found out, and when that happens it will be over and your reputation in the greater kink community may be seriously tarnished, because femdoms talk to each other. So think before declaring something a limit, and try to articulate what type of limit it is for you.

The other area of selfishness for slaves involves the things you need and want in a relationship. It can be very difficult for a would-be slave, or a slave currently serving, to make statements about what he wants, because he sees it as being inappropriately selfish or, worse, topping from the bottom. Just stating that you like to do a certain activity isn't topping from the bottom as long as you accept your owner's decision on that activity. It becomes a serious problem when you have a checklist of activities you "must" have, or have scripted out a scenario that you demand be followed. All fine for a bottom in a scene, perhaps, but is it really how a slave should be behaving? We don't think so.

However, someone who truly wishes to serve and submit is going to struggle with giving out his list of needs and wants. We have found two approaches that work to help slaves be more positively selfish in this regard. First, when she asks what you want, think of her request as a command to be obeyed. When you are asked what you like to do or what you need, take a moment before you reflexively say, "Nothing, Mistress," and find a way to express your feelings in a way that feels less like a demand to you. Some slaves add phrases like, "if it pleases you," at the end of their statements about needs and wants. Others bring gifts or toys with them that reflect what they enjoy and just add them to the equipment the dominant has. This is what Fox did early on in our dynamic, but TammyJo pushed things by asking him, "What is this for?" and waiting until he could tell her in some fashion before using anything.

You may not always be asked about your needs and wants as a slave. In fact, it is a more common experience for an owner to get into a comfortable flow and just not think of checking in as long as things seem to be working well on her end of things. Finding a good time to tell your Mistress what you wish could happen more often or what you feel is missing from the dynamic is not being selfish if, once again, you respect her decision. A good way to do this is to first get permission to speak to her. Then praise something she is doing right and make a statement about something that you really miss or really like when she does it. Does this mean you'll definitely get what you want or need? Sadly, no, but at least you put out the information, and now it's up to her to exercise her authority and make a decision. Over time, it should become easier to talk about such things. Fox went from bringing a backpack with bondage equipment in it to just being able to say, "I really need to be mummified soon, Mistress." You see, Fox kept hoping that bondage play would be offered spontaneously. Feeling that it was not his place as a submissive to ask for what he wanted, he invited disappointment.

Selfishness is even more difficult for many owners. One of the worst lies we are taught as women is that it is wrong to be selfish. From the moment we are born, it seems, we are trained to think of others, and to be aware of other people's moods, needs, and desires, often putting our own life on hold for husband, children, or parents. And yet, being the dominant, being the owner of a slave, is an innately selfish position. You are doing this for yourself; the world you create may in fact revolve around your experiences, your wishes, and your will. That contradiction can be very difficult for a woman to work around.

A lot of women react by not being selfish. They take on the role of a mother instead of that of an owner. They take on the role of a teacher instead of that of Mistress. They spend so much time getting to know their submissive that they ignore their own desires. Then they complain about how there are no "truly submissive men" out there.

Before you can be loyal to yourself, to defend yourself, you have to know what is good for you and what is harmful to you. That means taking the time to explore things for yourself first and foremost. That is one way of being selfish. Selfish isn't negative; it is merely looking out for number one, who happens, by the way, to be you.

Oh, yes, it is you. How can you possibly take care of anyone else if you can't take care of yourself? How can you teach someone else if you are ignorant? How can you fulfill someone's desire to serve if you have no idea how you want to be served? How can you love someone until you've experienced the primary love and acceptance of yourself?

There are women out there who are selfish in a bad sense of that word. They lie, they manipulate, they focus solely on material matters, and they treat their partners as if they were disposable. They constantly tell anyone who will listen how wonderful they are and denigrate anyone who looks at the world in a different fashion. Perhaps they're not as confident as they appear and are really narcissistic, which means they're trying to cover up their weaknesses by overemphasizing their strengths? Or perhaps they lack the ability to empathize because of some trauma in their lives? They might sound all hot, with the "kneel, worm" attitude they spout, but how many of them have stable, healthy, long-term slaves they've lived with and loved with for years upon years? You know the type of people we're referring to in this paragraph. They make everyone around them who isn't under their sway uncomfortable.

Part of being selfish in a positive fashion involves stopping for at least a few seconds before you make any decision to ask whether that choice is going to be the best for you — not just for this moment, but for the foreseeable future. It means taking any decision and adding yourself into the equation. For example, TammyJo has to make decisions about extra hours at Fox's job every now and again, because it's part of her authority to decide how he spends his time away from her. A huge part of that decision is his financial well-being and his health, both mental and physical. However, she also takes a moment to consult her calendar. Does she need him or want him on that Saturday? If she has made plans for them, the answer to the overtime is "No," because she believes that honoring their plans is showing commitment to their relationship and being loyal to what she needs, consistent time with him. Since she can make these sorts of choices financially, when he's had steady work for an entire week, and careerwise, because Fox is out to his supervisor at work, it is a positive selfishness. If the money were needed because we were behind on bills, if she had nothing planned, or if he really missed work, it could be a negative selfishness that could have ramifications for months to come.

A common complaint we see in online communities and hear from male submissives is that dominant women push themselves too hard and seem unable to delegate. Being selfish is also about paying attention to yourself so you aren't going at 110% all the time. Think about it. 110% might work for a short time to get you through a crisis, but it can't last. Always trying to be superwoman or never getting help to do your chores or handle your responsibilities means you're going to burn out. That will eventually bring mental or physical harm to yourself. A man who only wants to bottom or submit from time to time may not care, but a man who wants to be your slave wants to care about you. Remember our discussion about the internal conflicts male submissives can feel between their desire to serve and be controlled compared to their "man's job" of taking charge and taking care? Thinking about what you want and need first and foremost gives him a chance to experience all of that at the same time. While it can be a constant struggle to let go of your "I can do it all" attitude, when you do you'll be amazed at how relaxed and healthy you can feel.

How do you do this? Here is some advice from TammyJo, who is definitely fighting the positive fight to be more selfish. For all her claims of all of this being about her first and foremost, let's be honest; she pushes herself hard, and she expects perfection from herself even under circumstances she cannot control. These are the steps she's taken to try to be more selfish.

- *Admit that you have a problem, and see the damage you are doing to yourself physically and emotionally. Massage therapy was a huge part of this process, for TammyJo, because it forced her into her body once a month and helped her learn what it was like to just let go and feel instead of always thinking and planning ahead.*
- *Keep a journal of your desires and wants. While this was part of the process of designing a contract and training program, it*

really began as an attempt to improve her own life. It started off as mostly vague ideas and feelings, but over the years and with repeated practice she's been able to get more specific.

- Talk to your partner about how you feel. No, I don't mean that vague emotional talk and checking in that women can be famous for. I mean real communication, with specifics about what you need or want and what they have done or could do to help you get to the emotional condition you know is better for you. This is scary. He might think less of you for admitting you are afraid or you feel uncertain. Never forget, though, that being the dominant here means having the courage to stand up for you both, and that begins with you.

- Stop and think before reacting. This is very tough if you have the idea that being the owner equals knowing it all. You don't, and you can't, so work on admitting that and instead think of it as information gathering. To make the best decision you need to gather and weigh everything, right? You owe it to yourself and your slave to stop, ask questions, get a breath of fresh air, or whatever you need before you react. Just reacting without thinking is not being in control of yourself, and it is very hard to control another if you aren't at least trying to improve your self control.

- Start with little things. If it's hard for you to accept help, start getting "help" before you really need it. TammyJo has always been protective of her kitchen; she watched Fox like a hawk the first time he made her a sandwich. But she told him to do it and made herself watch from the edge of the kitchen. Thank goodness, because there are times when illness or obligations outside the household were made much easier by the knowledge that Fox could prepare a decent meal.

- Let yourself relax and feel served. Try this with yourself first by just setting aside some time when you read a book or take a bath without interruptions. See how great that makes your mind and body feel? Now set aside a few moments in your play time and just tell your slave to "please you." You did train him, right? You have communicated your feelings when you've played before, correct? Allow him an opportunity to just give for a few minutes.

If that feels good then extend those minutes into half hours or entire scenes every now and then. Then take that attitude, your newly felt power and authority out and apply it to everyday life. Instruct him on how you'd like him to dress or when certain chores will be done. Then, after he's practiced the new skill, allow him to show you his commitment by performing without a reminder. This can be very challenging if you or he believes that obedience is reactive, but as we'll discuss next, nothing could be further from the truth, and it forms the submissive's part of the foundations for your successful femdom lifestyle.

Obedience

Obedience. Time and again we see online and hear at munches that what a slave owes to his owner is obedience, period. What does that mean, how does it bolster your M/s dynamic, and how can it threaten your relationship?

Obedience can be simply doing what you are told when you are told. Although this can be very difficult for a man who has been raised by his family and society to be the one doing things, doing what you are told can be very erotic for most submissives and slaves. At that moment you release all of your worries about figuring out what to do and simply act. For owners it is a tremendous emotional rush to see or hear someone simply do as they are told.

It is almost the exact opposite of how things work in vanilla relationships, where we barter with each other, set up lists of chores, hope our partner performs their tasks, and sometimes even argue for years about why something hasn't been done that we "agreed" would be done. This is a situation that can easily arise between equals or between people who haven't taken the time to figure out what tasks are best suited to each person. It can also arise when both people are thinking more about self and immediate desire than what is good for the couple or the family. In an M/s dynamic you should both be supporting the authority arrangement: and thus, when the owner says, "jump," the slave jumps.

Sometimes obedience is part of play or sex, and when that is the case is it undeniably exciting for everyone. Other times obedience focuses on mundane tasks that are boring or dirty or time-consuming. Being obedient at these times is one reason why you should keep your commitment to your owner, and her giving you these tasks is one way she exercises her authority and is being selfish for a while. If you find that all the mundane stuff is just not what you are looking for, we have a few harsh-sounding words: You probably aren't cut out to be a slave. You could be a wonderful bottom, but slavery means serving someone other than yourself to the best of your ability.

To help you cope with the drudgery that is an innate part of being a slave, try to focus on the results of your obedience. We'll bet she seems happier and the household runs more smoothly when you clean the bathroom or pick up some groceries. Also remind yourself that telling you to do these things may be difficult for her, especially if she used to do these particular chores before you came along. She's allowing you to serve her in very personal ways when she trusts you to take on tasks she's been doing for years and years. If you focus on her motivation and the effects the results of your obedience have on her, you'll find obedience and the tasks themselves more palatable.

It isn't unusual for slaves to really thrive on pleasing an owner in the most mundane ways, but, as the world of kink draws in more and more people, it also isn't terribly common. As an owner, when you find someone who is truly obedient, take a moment or two to acknowledge his good work and his positive attitude. You don't need to reward him; you don't even need to thank him each time he obeys, but a kind word is a great way to help him want to be more obedient.

Sometimes a Mistress will give an order that is utterly silly and seemingly pointless. TammyJo actually loves to do this — and often. It can range from suddenly saying, "dance," in the middle of a grocery store, to "smile" at home, to "walk around the table" at a munch. These are not moments of formal play time or a scene in the bedroom; these activities accomplish no necessary task, and yet these moments are very important to bolstering the authority structure you have. The reason is simple: Immediate obedience reinforces your roles and your mutual acceptance of them.

For dominants, this is the ultimate in positive selfishness, because giving a silly order is a pure exercise of your power and authority for you and you alone. It might be embarrassing for your slave to dance in the dairy aisle, but his doing it proves he trusts you to make a good decision. Describing the feeling is difficult, but it is like knowing you are the most sexy, intelligent, and amazing woman on the planet for a few minutes. When you are down, this can just brighten your entire day. When you feel uncertain or stressed, it can help you relax.

Obeying is also valuable to slaves personally as well. According to Fox, performing these often whimsical commands offers him the chance to show his power and skill to improve Mistress' mood. Over the years, the motivation for obeying these commands has become internalized to the point where it's mostly automatic, but when considering it more deeply, he believes it's also a matter of maintaining his honor with regard to our contract. Sometimes ... it's just fun. It can be difficult for an adult male in a patriarchal society to just be cute and silly without worrying about how it will be viewed by others. In this case, obeying gives him permission to behave "differently" while knowing that if anyone asks why, he can just smile and point in Mistress' direction.

Practice in giving commands and obeying can have important benefits as well should a dangerous situation arise. Imagine a mummified slave who has drifted off to sleep (something that can and has happened to Fox in the past). Now, suppose when he wakes up that he's disoriented by his confinement and doesn't remember what has happened to him. This could lead to a panicked struggle to get free which could send him toppling out of bed and onto the floor, resulting in injury. A slave who is trained to reflexively obey would only need to hear "Stop moving" to avert danger. We've heard stories from other M/s couples and families over the years about how immediate obedience has saved the lives of both the owner and the slave. So work on being silly in your orders and on being immediate with your obedience to even the weirdest commands. You'll have fun, and you'll increase your levels of trust by showing your commitment over and over again to each other.

There are times when even the best of slaves will find it difficult to obey. We aren't talking about commands that go against your morals or ethics or that endanger you here. We hope you took the time to get to know each other beforehand so you didn't pick an owner who would issue such orders. There are simply times and situations when obeying seems very, very hard. This usually means times when a submissive is sick or exhausted from a day at work, but it can also just be when a command is given while the slave is intensely focused on another task. Such is the case sometimes with Fox. Occasionally, Mistress will ask for a glass of water or request a hug while Fox is in the middle of a computer task where interruption could mean the loss of hours of work. In such a situation, Fox will acknowledge the call with a "Yes, Mistress" to confirm that he has heard, and follow it with a request for a minute (or five) while explaining the reason for the delay. Mistress knows that if she were to refuse the extension Fox would comply, but she realizes that he would probably be distracted by the important task instead of being focused entirely on her request, which is what she really wants. Another example would be when Fox steps in the door, worn out from a long day at work, and Mistress asks him to help her to prepare dinner.

He wants to sit down and have a soda and cool off, but instead he'll nod and proceed to the kitchen. One of these situations is of external importance, and the other involves immediate feelings.

Needs & Wants

You started down this journey of consensual slavery because it fulfilled some need or want you had inside as either the dominant or the submissive. While we'll get more into the realities of matching these needs and wants, we want to first define the different terms, discuss them briefly, and then dive into one of the biggest areas of potential conflict and reward in a femdom relationship: fetishes.

One of the trickiest steps you will need to take as you begin your journey into consensual slavery or ownership is figuring out the differences between what you need and what you want. Why is this tricky? Well, aside from the basic human needs we all have, wants can masquerade as needs, and one person's want may be another person's need. A psychologist both Fox and TammyJo studied in college and whom they respect, Abraham Maslow, developed a schema for looking at a person's needs, and today experts call it "Maslow's Hierarchy of Needs." One reason his model works for us is that it places emphasis on what motivates a person to become the best he or she can become. We think a healthy M/s dynamic should also do this. Let's look briefly at his need categories and how they fit into the owner-slave relationship.

Physiological needs are those basic things that we need to survive as human beings. These include food, water, air, and sleep. If you don't have a way to procure these basics, there is no way you can focus on anything else; your life is basically a daily struggle to survive. Pooling your resources within an M/s dynamic can be a way to increase your ability to have these needs met. Closely related are the security needs, which include things like a steady income, healthcare, shelter, or a sense of safety from anyone who might harm you or take away the resources you need to fulfill your other needs. Needs like these are one reason why human beings form societies to begin with. Having either two producers or one producer with someone else to guard the materials acquired or created has been a principal way families have survived since the beginning of time. As we'll discuss later in this book when we talk about how this all works from day to day, who occupies which role depends on you, your abilities, and your other needs. There is no more reason for the slave to stay at home than for him to be the one with the job that pulls in the majority of money for a couple.

It is a matter of what you both want and what the circumstances around you make feasible. Some of these needs are addressed by the larger society in which you live, which has laws and law enforcement agents to help offer you security, or perhaps an educational system that teaches us to respect each other's property and bodies. Feeling safe requires that you trust someone, and trust is one of the building blocks for any relationship.

Next are the social needs that each of us has. Think of these as feeling connected to others and feeling valued by others. This need may be what drove you to venture out to your first munch or speak up on a web forum or answer an ad in the personals section of your local paper. We all need to feel like we belong in some fashion. Obviously creating a femdom relationship is one way to feel connected, but it is doubtful that one relationship can fulfill all your social needs. While it is common for people in a new relationship to spend a great deal of time with each other, it is not normal for a dominant to utterly restrict a submissive's interactions with others. That's a setup for an abusive relationship, not an M/s one. At the same time, your need for social connection can vary greatly. TammyJo loves to be around like-minded people in face-to-face situations; the Internet is a poor substitute for this. Fox, on the other hand, thrives more online and finds that his stress levels rise in face-to-face meetings. Yet both have ways of feeling connected to others, and both give each other the time and opportunity to make those connections.

Once those three types of needs are met, Maslow's theory states that a human being will then look to have her or his esteem needs met. What are esteem needs? These are like a more personal social need, because they require you to feel that you have personal worth, that you get social recognition, and that you have accomplishments you can feel proud of and which are valued by others. You get this not only from interacting with others but also by valuing yourself. A lot of people get stuck at this level. Not everyone is going to like you, you won't always win or succeed, and every one of us feels down at times. Having a partner who can encourage you is great — either a Mistress or a slave can do that — but your partner isn't God; they can't make things work out wonderfully for you every time. Some people just seem to be unlucky, unskilled, or perhaps chronically depressed. Being around those people is draining, even for the most upbeat and positive person. If you find you are having difficulty getting your esteem needs met, then you need to start evaluating your relationships, including the one with yourself.

Finally, if all four of those types of needs are met, Maslow defined what he called the self-actualizing needs, which he considered the highest need that we each should aim for. We agree with the idea that we should each be working toward or exercising at this level. What are self-actualizing needs, anyway? These include self-awareness, which in terms of BDSM can mean understanding your needs and wants, your limitations and your abilities in an honest fashion. They also include working toward bettering yourself and feeling less worried about what others think of your decisions and actions. Of course, in an M/s relationship you will be concerned about your partner, but being at the self-actualizing level means you are confident enough to use your power to make your relationship work as well as self-aware enough to have picked an appropriate owner or slave to begin with.

If these are needs, then how do they differ from wants, which can be found in any of Maslow's categories? Think of it this way: you need certain nutrients in your food and drink to be healthy, but your desire for chocolate or caviar is a want. You need protein, but whether you get it in beef, fish, or beans is a want (as well as a reflection of your economic means and geographical location). Similarly, we each have a need to be secure, to connect with others, and to feel valuable, but whether you get it through a traditional marriage, a religious order, or a femdom relationship may be more of a want.

One way to sort out your needs from your wants within your relationship is to start keeping track of which types of interactions make you feel best. Break down a good scene and try to determine what specifically made you feel the safest, the most valued, the most beneficial, or the most true to yourself. Was the fact that you were bound with ropes really what was important, or was the fact that you knew your partner could be trusted more important? Is his picking up your shoes with his teeth the thing that really made you feel strong, or is it the fact that you know he will obey you that gives you a sense of fulfillment? The odds are that the specifics of how something is done are not as important as the action itself or the motivation behind it. You can have many different ways to achieve the same goal or get your needs met; the wants are those ways.

We're sorry we can't give you more specific guidelines to figuring out your own list of needs and wants. That is very personal and may change over the years. We can say with 100% certainty that the more you know about your own needs and wants, the better owner or slave you'll make, and the more comfortable you'll be communicating them once you are in a relationship. A person's needs are not negotiable, ever, but how they are achieved — their wants — may be. If someone's wants differ too much from your own, that may spell trouble in the future. One of the areas we've noticed that can have the greatest degree of variation is in the area of fetishes.

Fetishes: A Special Type of Want

We're sure you've heard the word "fetish" before. There's a clinical definition of the term, and there's popular culture's widespread use of the term. In the clinical sense, a fetish is an object that is required for sexual arousal and satisfaction. In other words, without the object you can't get hard or wet, and you certainly can't orgasm. Often this is considered a problem, because it separates the person from other people, thus inhibiting their ability to connect with others sexually and often emotionally. From TammyJo's viewpoint this is a terrible thing for an owner to have to deal with, because it strips you of the ability to be as creative with your partner, since you must cater to his fetish. You both become enslaved to the fetish object, if the interest can be classified as a fetish by a mental healthcare professional.

The more general term "fetish" can be seen as a tool in a mistress-slave relationship. This is the way the term is more often used in the BDSM communities. Since Fox has done a few presentations about fetishes in BDSM, we're going with his definitions. Fetishes are more like preferences or wants that greatly enhance the experience through sensory stimulation, increased comfort and sense of safety, etc.

With this broader definition in place, we believe that most people have fetishes to some degree. Even within this general definition, though, there are two types of fetishes that we see time and again in BDSM: object fetishes and relationship fetishes — or tangible and intangible fetishes, if you want to sound more scientific. Let's look at both types and how they can be used to empower your relationship.

Object Fetishes. An object fetish is usually what you think of when you think "fetish." This attraction to an inanimate object or material can be for almost anything you can imagine, ranging from an item of clothing, such as shoes, to a type of fabric, like lace, to a household item, like a brush, to a very specific object, like the back seat of a red Cadillac convertible. The attraction can appeal to several senses. It may be the look of a color, the feel of a fabric, the scent of an object, or perhaps even the taste or sound it makes. The most important point for you to remember as the owner or slave is that this object helps arouse your partner or yourself, but it is merely one of several ways you can get reactions and get off. Thus you can use it creatively, if you choose.

Many people have multiple object fetishes that appeal to several senses. Let's take an example. You could have a partner who loves the feel of velvet, adores the look of a corset on someone else, and is aroused by the scent of lilacs. You can choose to use one, two, or all three of these from time to time with your partner to enhance his enjoyment of the moment.

The power to use object fetishes is not limited to the dominant, even though it often appears that way in pornography, erotica, and even discussions at kinky gatherings. Let's say your partner likes the look of a smooth face, the feel of silk, and the smell of cinnamon. You as the slave could maintain a clean shave, invest in some silk shirts or pants, and find a cinnamon candle or even do some baking. There, you've just turned on your Mistress as easily as she turned you on by using your own object fetishes.

Between Fox and TammyJo, he is the one with the object fetishes. No, we aren't going to discuss his fetishes specifically, for a very good reason. TammyJo worked to learn about these, and she wants to keep her authority to use them to herself. If you want to learn what they are, maybe he'll share some with you, if you get to know him. We will, however, hint at them in the forthcoming section about using fetishes in your relationship.

Relationship Fetishes. This type of fetish is something we talked about for a few years when Fox was getting his minor in psychology. Because he has object fetishes, Fox thought that was the only type of fetish. But after consideration of what appeared to be TammyJo's fetish for collars on other people, we realized that the psychology of the collar and the motivation behind it was TammyJo's fetish – thus was born the idea of a relationship fetish. We both have relationship fetishes, which means that certain types of personal relationships appeal to us highly, so highly that they are a guarantee to turn us on and generally are a nice help to getting us off. Sometimes these can be quite important, forming the foundation of a particular relationship. However, as a long-term couple, we have to connect on a variety of levels simply to deal with life – so our relationship fetishes stay outside the realm of a clinical fetish.

You've heard of relationship fetishes, but you probably just think of them as different roles people choose. Queen-knight, Mommy-baby, owner-puppy, lady-sissy, captor-captive, sultan-harem slave, and teacher-student are just a small sample of the multitude of roles in femdom dynamics. So if you masturbate while thinking about being a Queen or about being a puppy, you may have a relationship fetish.

These sorts of fetishes can be great fun to play with, but, unlike object fetishes, they can be tricky to use. The reason is that this type of fetish is about a relationship, and that goes beyond a mere role to include a scenario or situation and perhaps even a personality type for the partner with this type of interest. Just putting on the pirate garb so you can get captured by your partner in a naval officer's uniform won't cut it. You have to act the part, and this can get tricky for many people.

One reason why it's tricky is that too often we associate role-playing with either the profession of acting or the childhood stage of life. We are adults, and very few of us consider ourselves actors. We'll talk more about how to use relationship fetishes in the next part of this subsection.

Figuring out what your relationship fetishes are is a bit complicated. You might imagine yourself as a cat because you saw lots of cats in cartoons, but what exactly about being a cat turns you on? Before you can explain your relationship fetish to anyone else, you have to understand it yourself. You can do this by reflecting and manipulating what you do privately.

First, write down those fantasy scenarios that keep playing in your mind when you masturbate. You may discover that you have a few different ones with different roles or characters you identify with. What is common between the Queen and the Warrior, between the Puppy and the Baby? If you can determine that, you have a good chance of understanding your relationship fetish but also what type of general dynamic works for you. For example, you might discover you want to be in charge, but sometimes in an active and sometimes in a passive way. You may find out that you like being praised sometimes for what you do and sometimes simply for being there. You may also discover contradictory things, but that's OK. Human beings are complex, and we should expect everything about ourselves to be complex, even our fetishes.

Next, try changing the scenery and the customs in your fantasies, but using those commonalities you've discovered. TammyJo learned that she functions best in a relationship when she is clearly the one in charge because every single one of her fantasies involved her having authority over one or more people. It didn't matter if she was a spaceship captain or sexy teacher or the leader of a tiny country; the details didn't mean as much as the underlying relationship. This fantasy work, coupled with TammyJo's natural drive to be in charge and her extreme distaste for taking orders or following, helped her accept that this relationship fetish went beyond the fetish level to that of Need, which we discussed earlier. The fantasies are extremes of that Need, and so we can play around with the idea by setting aside time when she exercises more authority over a wider range of activities. Luckily Fox likes just following orders and "relaxing" from time to time, so it works out well.

However, some relationship fetishes are best left in the realm of role-playing. For example, TammyJo says, "I've learned that my relationship fetishes often involve rescuing people. At first I thought this was just related to imagining myself buying a slave at an auction, but then I realized that this was the same situation I was in when I imagined myself as an Amazon warrior claiming the abused captive or the wealthy professional picking up the street punk." With this knowledge we can play out various roles for fun. But building your relationship as the person who always rescues may be very stressful over time. You will need help yourself at some point — again, that is just part of being human — but if you see yourself as that White Knight, you may never let yourself ask for, demand, or even acknowledge that you need assistance. Being a goddess is a nice job, but only if you are a goddess, and we're fairly sure that you aren't.

Fetish and Empowerment. Using your partner's fetishes to enhance your dynamic and your own power does not mean stripping power away from him. If you use the fetishes in positive ways, in creative ways, you are actually sending a message that you value your partner's desires, because you have learned what their fetishes are and have invested time and thought in using them. You can, of course, construe this as your having power over or manipulating the other person. That is fun to play with but for a long-term relationship probably not terribly healthy. The last thing you want to do is harm your partner's ability to enjoy his fetishes or limit your own power by making him dependent upon them, resulting in a clinical fetish. We don't know about you, but we like our power to be creative and inspiring to each other, so we keep it varied in intensity and frequency.

Learning about a partner's fetishes, be they tangible or intangible, can be done in two ways. The direct approach works best if you have been in a relationship for some time. This is simply because there is often a social dirtiness attached to admitting you have a fetish. In pop culture, fetishes are viewed as silly or destructive. Neither need be the case, but this portrayal of them can be difficult to get past psychologically. Even a few years ago it was difficult for us to tell each other some of our fantasies and the fetishes involved in them, because they seemed so extreme to us. We each worried that we might be rejected for these "weird ideas."

Take TammyJo's interest in ignoring consent, an innate part of many of her relationship fetishes. This is not something she would ever do in reality; being a survivor of sexual violence herself makes her all too aware of the harm that having one's consent ignored has on a person forever. At the core, this fetish is an extension of being in control and a rejection of how she was raised to care for others before herself. Luckily within BDSM we have something called consensual-nonconsensual dynamics. This can be done on an ongoing basis, where the dominant assumes that consent is given unless it is actively withdrawn, or in a role-play or scene, where the words "no" or "stop" are ignored for a short period of time. Telling Fox she had these desires, though, went against everything he knew she held dear. There was a chance he would withdraw his consent to be her slave and walk out the door. Once she shared it, though, scary as it was, he expressed surprise that she had trouble sharing it, because it seemed rather obvious to him that she had these desires, given the scenarios and fantasies she has. Sometimes your partner knows before you do.

That isn't always the case. A former partner of TammyJo's fetishized being a woman, and that, too, involved risk when he told TammyJo about it. While she may be a feminist, she does not have deep understanding of people who want to be a different sex, race, or other things she considers innate. Unlike Fox's reaction to TammyJo's fetish for nonconsensuality, TammyJo was very surprised to learn about this desire, because she always considered her partners to be androgynous rather than heavily gendered. She didn't and doesn't understand this partner's fetish to become a woman — and it was a fetish, since there was no desire to make such a change permanent — but she didn't reject this former partner because of it either. Instead it led to rare role-playing scenarios where her partner would be dressed as a woman and they'd go shopping, for example, without the D/s overtones. This is an example of how sharing your fetish may not result in getting everything you want but also may not go to the extreme you fear.

Hearing about a fetish can be challenging on several levels. First, if it's an object, you may start believing your partner finds the fetish more important than you. As long as we are talking about the general fetish and not the clinical definition, that shouldn't be the case. Second, you may feel that knowing about the fetish requires that you use it. This is a bigger challenge, because in order for both of you to do the work required to power your relationship, you both must get something positive from it on a consistent basis. Just remember that you have the power to interpret and use those fetishes in a way that is beneficial to you both. If you have a negative reaction, be honest about that, and don't pretend you can go along with it. If you have a neutral reaction, then you owe it to your partner and yourself to explore a bit. Perhaps you can couple one of your partner's fetishes with one of your own. For instance, when we role-play that we're at an auction, one buying (TammyJo) and one being bought (Fox), he's usually garbed in appropriate clothing or bondage gear.

You can help your partner hear about your fetishes with a more open mind by choosing your approach carefully. Don't spring several at once. Pick a time when your partner is feeling comfortable, relaxed and above all safe in the relationship. Don't expect them to fulfill your fetishes that moment or the next day. In fact, don't expect them to fulfill it at all. Give the information, answer the questions, and then give your partner a chance to try things out. This is difficult, because if your partner just isn't interested they may never want to give it a try. Don't give up, but try a different approach the next time you tell them about the fetish. Try asking them about a fantasy, situation or fetish they might have first, then see if you can do something to fulfill that. Lay the positive groundwork so you have fertile ground to sow your own fetish upon.

Ultimately you may find yourself in a relationship where your partner rejects all of your fetishes. We think this is probably rare if you have taken the time to approach carefully and waited until you are in a good, safe place in your relationship. Nevertheless, the possibility exists, and when it does happen you have to ask yourself some hard questions — questions which are exactly like the ones we discussed when we talked about Needs and Wants. This is going to sound cruel, but in the end you may need to end your relationship to get your Needs and Wants, and these can include fetishes, met. That has to be your choice, a choice you are always free to make, but it means ending the relationship — not simply withdrawing or retaliating against your partner in some fashion.

So we can't promise that you will get everything you want if you take the direct approach to telling your partner about your fetish. We can say that it is unlikely after several years together that your partner will simply dump you for sharing one fetish at a time, no matter how dark it is. If they do, how much of a partner were they in the first place? We can promise that unless you are willing to share, none of your fetishes, fantasies, or desires will be met.

Another way to uncover your partner's fetishes or share your own is the subtle way. When you begin your relationship, and even during the first few years, you'll learn more about your partner's fetishes through observation and questions. Does your partner sigh happily when you wear something or say a certain word? Does your partner smile a bit wider when you watch a particular scene in a movie? After observing several times you can search for more information, but be sure you do it in a gentle fashion without making any statements that might sound like a judgment.

Here are some examples: "I noticed that you watch me a lot when I brush my hair, and then you seemed to really enjoy the scene in that movie where the man was being spanked by a hairbrush. I'm thinking of using my hairbrush on your bottom soon." Then watch for a reaction. If it's positive, experiment. Look for reactions when you spank him using a hairbrush, but also when you just rub it on his arm or have him brush your hair with it. What is he interested in? Pain, the brush itself, the feeling of a particular area of the brush? After several such attempts, you should be able to figure out what he likes and incorporate that into the ways you interact with him.

Voila! You've just read your partner's mind. Or that is what it will seem like to him, because without asking for direct information (which may make him shy or defensive), you have figured out one of his fetishes, and you can now use it to increase your mutual pleasure. Remember, this course of action can be used by submissives too — so don't feel left out or think you have no work to do, guys.

If your partner has more experience or education about herself, she may just share some of her fetishes with you as you discover other ones. Some of these are so common — shoes, rubber, collars — that they will be easy to share. However, objects may hide relationships, so you'll still need to observe and experiment to learn what makes your partner tick. You may also learn that it only takes a word or a simple flash of an object to get a big reaction, and this increases your repertoire tremendously. This happens all the time in our house. There are several words and phrases that TammyJo can say where Fox will respond by gasping or dropping his eyes in a particular fashion. These little actions and reactions need not lead to sex or scenes, but can merely serve as a reassurance to you and your partner that you're both in this owner-slave dynamic for the long haul.

That's what we have to say about finding and using fetishes, but what is your job if your partner is using your fetishes? First, be encouraging. If your partner is going to the effort of wearing that silk shirt, make your touches a bit more intense. If your partner is using a term you find exciting, smile a bit wider. Sometimes you may not be in the mood, so pretend it turns you on. Yup, that's right: pretend. Exaggerate your feelings. This is a lot like smiling or humming happily when you feel sad and discovering that it actually lifts your emotions a bit. Exaggeration is especially important if your partner has limited skills with reading body language and tone of voice (this is more common for men, but not rare for women either).

Second, don't be greedy. Remember this is about your dynamic, not about your fetishes — not even the relationship ones. Enjoy it when your partner uses a fetish for you both, but don't expect it all the time, and don't complain if days go by without that pair of pink pumps or the playful whimper. If using your fetishes starts to feel like a job, we know for a fact your partner will start resenting having to use them, because you are curbing her creativity and limiting the ways he can serve. Plus, if you use your fetish all the time you may find it creates less and less excitement for you as your body and mind become used to the stimulus. Value the thrill when you see your fetish or engage with your partner in those ways. Part of the fun is in that thrill, so don't dilute it by overusing it.

Finally, remember to reciprocate. The odds are very high that your partner has fetishes, too. Learn what they are and try to use those. If the preferences and desires are not quite at the fetish level, and they aren't a guaranteed way to get arousal, then use those wants to show your partner that you paid attention and care about them. When your partner feels valued, they will do things to make you feel valued in return. If they don't, you may need to rethink your consent to be in that dynamic at all.

One final thought about fetishes. Do not call attention to the fact that you have just been so generous as to fulfill your partner's desire to see the color black, smell chocolate, or feel rubber. The hardness of his cock or the wetness of her pussy is a sure sign that you have indeed done something they like. Let them react naturally or encourage you through their reactions. Don't demand a pat on the head. That's needy for a submissive, undignified as a dominant, and unattractive for both.

Privacy

In most of the western world, for all our social networking, gossiping, and love of reality TV, most of us have the expectation that we will have some privacy in our lives. In fact, emotionally we probably need to have some time just to ourselves and some information about ourselves that we don't want to share. When you enter into any type of relationship you lose some of your privacy. This can be a matter of merely being together, sharing space with another person. It can be a result of the communication you need to have in order to make things work smoothly. It can also be a reflection of your personality and your past dictating how much time alone you need or want.

This is another of those issues that is constantly debated in the M/s and D/s communities, both online and offline. Extremes of privacy can range from someone who must be in their owner's constant presence to someone who is locked in a full-body rubber suit and isolated from the rest of the world. These extremes sound erotic to many people, but in reality neither extreme will probably last for very long. There are just physical things you must do to live that might prove too challenging to maintain in that rubber suit all the time with no breaks at all. As obedient as he may seem, having someone with you 24/7 can start to feel very uncomfortable for even the most narcissistic dominant unless she truly stops seeing her slave as her partner and only as an object. We're giving advice for how to have a successful relationship between two people, not a person and a table.

People vary greatly in how much privacy they need and want, and even in what privacy means to them. Some people share what seem to be the most intimate details of their lives with perfect strangers while others only talk about vague, general matters. Some of us want to be around a lot of people all the time, while others value solitude. Most of us lie somewhere in the middle, happy to share a lot with a limited number of people and wanting to spend regular time with either the same group or another group of people. If you both have the same idea about how much you need to share about your lives and thoughts and how much time you want to spend together, then this section won't be of much help to you. Be happy you found a good match in this area. The odds are, though, that there are some differences between you two (or three, or however many people are a part of your M/s dynamic). While it would be easy to say that you just adjust to whatever the owner wants, real life does not work smoothly if that is your only option.

Fox is a much more private person than TammyJo. Think about it. As a college professor, as a published author and activist, she can hardly be especially private. Fox will use pseudonyms and avatars in his interactions online, whereas TammyJo is usually just TammyJo. She has a website to flaunt her work and hopefully generate more fans and more invitations to groups and events, while Fox doesn't even have a site for his web design business because he receives enough clients based on word of mouth. She has no problem telling her friends and co-workers in detail about everything going on in her life, and she can chat with a group of strangers fairly easily. Fox usually keeps all but the most major developments in his life to himself and finds it difficult to socialize with large groups of people he doesn't know.

A further irony is that TammyJo went from taking and teaching classes and being surrounded by colleagues and students all the time… to a career which has her by herself most of the week. Fox, on the other hand, went from living alone with more or less complete autonomy… to sharing a house with two other people and spending most of the week working alongside and supervising teams of people. At the end of the day, their need for privacy and alone time can be completely at odds.

These differences could have been a recipe for disaster except for one thing. TammyJo is actually not sharing what she considers very private information, and Fox actually loves attention and being the center of it. So while we look very different (and we are quite different), it isn't 180 degrees' difference between us. We can agree, for example, that there are some things we won't share in this book. As much as we want all of you to benefit from our experiences and struggles, some things we only discuss with our other partner or very close, personal friends. Other things we just want to keep between the two of us, because we feel they strengthen our M/s and our affection for each other.

But we did have to work out the differences we do have. The biggest one of these was time spent in close physical contact. Remember how we said you can't just fall back on what the Mistress wants? The reason is that even the most attentive slave is going to feel pressure or loneliness if his own needs for time alone or with someone are not met at least partway. That's just a natural human reaction; it has nothing to do with being more or less submissive. When we don't get what we need or want, we feel slighted, we feel hurt, or we feel like something isn't quite right. At the same time, you did both enter into this lifestyle with informed mutual consent. And the fact is that M/s is not an egalitarian relationship. Someone has more authority and may have more power here, so that person, the owner, is going to get a bit more in any compromise than the enslaved.

Fox likes to be close to TammyJo physically, but he has a job where he has to deal with people he doesn't necessarily like all day, five days a week. When he gets home she often require his services to help make dinner, set the table, or whatever. Of course he obeys, though there are times he'll tell her that he's had a terrible day and could really use a break, then hopes that her decision will be good for them both. As a slave he really just can't say "No" to her orders, even if they might be worded as requests. In fact, that's one of the rules in our long contract. But he has the responsibility to give her information, and she has a responsibility to think about her decisions.

FOUNDATIONS OF OWNER/SLAVE DYNAMICS

One way she might deal with his need for privacy and downtime is to send him off to his room between helping her and actual meal time. She often gives him an hour or two after dinner to just be by himself, then they watch something on TV together, play a game, just sit and talk, or do other things. Plus, he's more of a night person, so after the evening ritual, he tends to stay up doing whatever he needs or wants to do. No, she doesn't get to spend as much time with him as she'd like, but he also isn't as alone as he'd like, so it's a compromise for both of them.

There was a time when TammyJo owned and was training three people. That gave her four people, including her husband Tom, to balance into her life. She loved it, because it gave her all that time with close companions that she really craves. Sometimes people realize they aren't a great match — people move away for better jobs; life happens. She doesn't have her ideal household now. She and Fox both agree that they'd love to add at least one more slave to the family, but she isn't sure that adding someone would be a good idea while she feels that her career is in transition. The result is that both have to compromise far more on how much time they spend together than either would ideally like. Honestly, when the Mistress says, "I need you" to Fox, she gets him, so the bulk of the compromise is really on Fox's side.

How can he not feel tremendous resentment about this? According to Fox, before Faith and Anna departed, he could count on having certain blocks of uninterrupted time to himself, because Mistress would be occupied with one or the other of them. In this way, he could schedule activities that required intense concentration (such as classwork) or headspace (such as drawing) without worrying about being called on. When he became the only slave in the household, it did become harder for him to do these things, because he was the only one on call all the time. Add to this the challenge of having to fulfill the specialized roles vacated by his companions in addition to the ones he started with and agreed to, and soon the stress began to show. Over time, however, things began to settle into a more balanced state as our mutual expectations evolved to become more realistic and probable. Fox's role was now far broader, but he was no longer performing some of the incorporated roles with nearly the same frequency or intensity as Faith or Anna had.

Privacy also has to do with information, and this is a mutual problem that dominants and submissives can face even after years together. Because femdom is still so outside the social norm of behavior for men and women, there can be a lot of pressure to be perfect. This pressure can result in a fear about sharing information. However, one common mantra of BDSM that we do strongly agree with is that you must have good communication to make this work. It takes practice to tell your partner how you feel and what you're thinking — repeated practice, sometimes years of it. It also takes your partner asking questions — repeated questions, sometimes over years. Furthermore, it takes empathy to keep that communication going. We mentioned empathy on the side of the owner earlier when we talked about Selfishness, but slaves need empathy too if they are going to fully serve their owners. When a partner shares her feelings, you have to control your gut-level reactions and just encourage her to keep talking, repeat that she has a right to feel that way, and reassure her that you're still her boy. The reverse is also true when a slave breaks through his fears and shares his private worries, desires, and past with an owner.

We recommend setting up a safe place or a safe space where you can share private conversations. This can be a physical space, like a particular room of your house, or a relationship space, where you both agree that what is about to be talked about will not be used in any negative way later on. This is often called being "out of scene" with each other, and it happens after a while as you simply get used to encouraging and sharing your private thoughts and feelings more and more.

Ultimately it is probably healthy for each of us to have some things we just keep to ourselves and some time we have to just be with ourselves. Finding a balance will take time, and you are going to make mistakes as you work to find it. Just remember that part of your commitment is to work through these things together, even if that means dropping the Mistress and slave roles for a while.

Play Time

Ah yes, play time, or scene time, SM, bondage, or making love. It's whatever you call that time you set aside to do the wonderful BDSM things that made you want to find a stable M/s relationship in the first place. In the porn novels, short stories, and films, you'd think it was non-stop floggings and orgasms, living in cages, and crushing cigarettes out on tongues. Real life isn't like that, but it can be like that for small periods of time — sometimes every day, in fact, though not 24/7.

Oh, we can hear it now: the online claims of, "No, no, I live in a cage all the time," but hey, they must have a computer in that cage, and are they "doing it" all the time if they have time to toss their claims of "true slavery" out on every site? We don't think that's very logical either, so let's talk about how you can schedule and incorporate playtime into your everyday life as a way to keep it all flowing smoothly.

Some couples make "dates" or set aside time each week or month when they have full scenes, including costumes, equipment, music, or hours of different activities. If you are in regular jobs and have good health and stable ways to make time alone together, you can go this route. The trick to making this "special" time stay special is to talk about it between sessions. Perhaps buy a new toy or a new CD. Get a new piece of clothing, or have a ritual you each follow an hour or a day before to prepare. The greatest danger with this weekly or monthly date is that it can start to feel like a chore and less like pleasure. If something should come up that you can't schedule around, you can also feel a deep sense of failure. Whatever you do, keep in mind that this is time for you both to reconnect on that level that helped introduce you to a possible lifetime.

Some couples have so much time that they can schedule daily scenes. The scenes here have to vary a great deal to stay fresh and to allow for any physical healing that might need to happen. Let's face it — some of us play hard when we play, and the bruises and sore muscles may need time to heal. One session may focus on bondage, the next on flogging, the next on sex, then next on verbal abuse, and so on. You have to keep it moving along, or you might find yourself having Monday as puppy play night and Wednesday as flogging evening over and over again. As long as you are both happy, that's cool, but the danger again is that it may start to feel like a chore, not pleasure.

Whenever we see people online or at workshops asking for suggestions about what they can do next to their partner, we discover they are playing on a very regular basis. Running out of ideas may sound funny, but it appears to be very common. If you take a hard look at the activities covered by BDSM it can seem like a dazzling array, but in reality it's a short list of related activities that you put a new twist or take on. Flogging, caning, and spanking: all of these are impact play. Handcuffs, mummification, and shibari: all of those are forms of bondage. And so on and so forth.

Remember how we talked about the dominant taking pieces of her submissive's desires and fetishes and using them in slightly different ways? This is something to keep in mind in any scene. It can be very easy to fall into the trap of the same old same old. 20 swats with your hand, then 20 with a leather strap, and a final 20 with a wooden paddle can feel comforting, but why not add a few more of one of these one night, just to see what happens? For Mistresses changing things can be scary, because now you can't really predict how your slave will react. That's why some folks use safewords even years into their M/s dynamic while others have signals or open communication. Honestly, while it can be reassuring to do that same old same old, it can also get boring. Boring can kill passion.

One way to keep things fresh is to make sure you attend demonstrations of activities, have friends in the BDSM community you can share stories with, and simply do a lot of reading books/stories or watching films where kink is a factor. We aren't saying you have to do everything you see or hear about, but keeping up to date can help your own imagination when it comes to spicing things up.

That's not a job only for the ladies. Slaves, too, need to do their bit to keep it interesting. Express your enjoyment of the scene, and help her relax so she can get into it by making sure all those mundane things in her life are cleared away before playtime. Repeatedly, sex study after sex study has demonstrated that women need to relax to have great orgasms. Think of a scene as a mental orgasm. You want her to get into it? You want her to be creative? Help make sure she isn't thinking about dishes or the car payment before she places that gag on you.

Depending on the rules of your M/s dynamic, slaves may also be free to bring new toys, new clothes, or new ideas directly into a scene. Here's a suggestion — don't bring it right to the scene. Many Mistresses with scheduled play time plan things out in advance. Surprising her with a new set of candles might seem romantic, or it can seem like an attempt to direct the scene or criticize what she had planned. Instead, give her things before a scheduled scene — a day or two before. A lot of women like gifts, but you need to make sure that what you give her is appropriate to how she plays and to the way your dynamic flows. If your Mistress isn't into rubber, giving her a rubber skirt risks offending her or feeling like topping from the bottom.

Also think of what you can wear yourself or what you can do yourself to keep things fresh. Perhaps a new shirt in her favorite color that she can order you to strip out of or take off of you herself will inspire her. Perhaps adding words to your usual grunts and moans during a beating would please her. Make the words equally about you — "You've made this boy's skin so hot, Mistress" — and about her — "You are so powerful, Lady." Compliments, sincere ones, are generally welcomed by all owners we've known, because it is a form of positive feedback that reassures us we are truly worthy of your submission and service.

You can also just incorporate play time into your everyday interactions. This is actually the route that TammyJo and Fox take most often, because life can be too unpredictable for regular play time. Fox never knows when she might spank his ass or push him up against a wall. TammyJo can't be certain if Fox is going to kneel right now for no reason or look at her and beg for something. This keeps things constant, but also off-kilter enough that it remains exciting. Also, exercising our desire for each other, the authority and the submission, keeps the M/s present in our mind beyond the rules, rituals, and protocols we use.

Play time is about keeping the passion that brought you together fresh, so find a way of making it a part of your life — every day, every week, every month, or whatever works best for you both. Yes, sometimes it will feel like a chore, but once you get started, once you take on the challenge to do or react differently in some fashion this scene, you should discover how rewarding it still is to focus solely on each other for an hour or more.

7

DAILY REALITIES: ADJUSTING & MAINTAINING THE DYNAMIC

Economic Realities

The difference between BDSM as portrayed in porn and BDSM in reality seems most stark when we look at economics. When you think of the famous fiction works by our leading leather authors, you see independently wealthy men and women with harems of slaves, and land they couldn't walk in a day even if they tried. That mirrors perfectly the life that Fox and TammyJo lead.

Not!

We bet it doesn't represent your life very well either.

Some of the BDSM world is indeed wealthy. There are people who live on estates and who have both hired servants and consensual slaves. People who can go to Paris at a moment's notice and who can buy a $1000 pair of shoes without a thought. We don't meet many people who fall into this category, but the ones we have met (those we know are real) all have high-paying jobs they have to do in order to earn that income. What seems like a sudden vacation in Paris may actually be squeezed in between meetings with clients or managers. The new shoes may be a result of a particularly good quarter, a way to celebrate. So even those people are thinking about their money at some level, even if we average people don't see it.

For the rest of us, paying off the mortgage or school loans is a monthly chore we have to do. We may be doing decently or even be well off. We can afford to go to a leather convention or a few of them each year. We have the income and time to go to a monthly munch in three different cities a few hours from us. We splurge on new toys a few times a year or get a signed copy of a book from a visiting author. Money isn't a huge stress, but when things happen like medical bills or the car needing to be repaired, we do have to stop and breathe for a few moments to remind ourselves that it's all manageable.

While some internal studies of BDSMers say that we tend to be more educated and have a higher income than the general population, there are plenty of kinky people who are living below the average income level. Given the cycle of economic conditions nationwide and worldwide, some of us may even face times of poverty, when we're threatened with the loss of our job or house. That level of stress can certainly kill a Mistress's desire to lead or a slave's determination to obey. It might not even be conscious but simply a reaction to needing to find a way to pay this bill now instead of finding time to play or planning for the next munch.

We think part of the stress that M/s can feel from economics reflects how financial matters are handled in your relationship from the very start. If one person has all of the responsibility for every transaction, then when economic matters take a dive, she or he is going to feel particularly stressed. One sad result can be a change from M/s to abuse as the stressed partner finds their ability to empathize or care lessened.

There is a repeated debate in the general BDSM community about whether or not play should ever happen when the top is angry. We think it is also a matter of feeling stress in general, really. In fact, if you can control your behavior and if you both work to lessen the stress, play can be a good way to relieve some tension. There have been times that TammyJo has just started issuing orders because she felt economic or work situations slipping from her grasp, and knowing someone was there who would follow her willingly felt great. There have been times that Fox has offered his body up to her hands and toys to help relieve stress as well, though that doesn't generally make her feel as unburdened as it might other people.

One obvious way to lessen the financial strain is to not allow one person to carry all of the responsibilities related to your family finances. The model in which the owner must control everything having to do with money, while the slave just stays home and waits around to serve, is not necessarily desirable. In fact, this very idea that the slave is cared for financially does not reflect how historical slavery has worked for millennia nor how slavery continues to work today in many parts of the world. Just because yours is a consensual relationship, that doesn't mean you have to become basically a parent and support your slave. You could have him support you, you could both work, you could both be in school, or whatever arrangement works best for you. There is no one right way to do this, but you both need to agree that whatever you choose is a good financial arrangement that lessens the economic stress on you both. A Mistress who is worried about money can't lead very well, and a slave who is worried about finances isn't going to be doing his best job.

Often both people must work, though in our household the guys work for a steady income while TammyJo writes freelance. To balance their economic contributions she takes on two primary financial tasks. First, she does the majority of the shopping, and she considers it a sign of a good owner and wife to think long-term when making purchases. She weighs price with nutrition, thinks about who will use what and how often it will get used, and keeps track of coupons. The second task she takes on is being the final word on big purchases. Raised in a much lower income group than either Fox or Tom, her husband, she has had to do more budgeting than either of them. In other words, she manages and directs the financial matters to a large degree in the household....

... But not all of them, because that could be burdensome. First, Fox does not have a legal stake in the current house we all live in. So he contributes enough money to cover the resources he uses, like electricity, gas, water, some food costs, and cable. The point is that as the slave he is not a burden of any type, and this is one way he avoids being a drag on us all financially. Sadly, he took a less than ideal job when he decided that being TammyJo's and part of this family was more important than a high-paying career, which he could have had coming out of college with a very good degree in physics. He is fairly frugal and has paid off his school loans already. Currently, besides his monthly expenses, he's saving up to help when we are ready to move on to our next home.

Yup, he's going to help buy the next house, and that might shock a lot of you reading this if you think that being a consensual slave means never owning anything. That could work, but most M/s couples we know and respect have taken the time to make sure each partner is financially invested in the relationship. That's invested, mind you, not dependent. There's a big difference. Of course, a lot of M/s couples go that extra step and get married, or perhaps they started off married, and thus legally they have certain shared financial responsibilities and rights.

If you can't get married or don't want to, because you believe that marriage is a very different relationship from M/s, then you have to find ways to make everything financially sound for you both. We do it by Fox's having a job and controlling his own finances, and we are planning to take that next step in the future with a house owned three ways. Any other step, such as legal contracts, we cannot give informed advice about. Find a lawyer who specializes in such matters. If you are too worried about legal costs, then you might want to consider your commitment to this dynamic. You have to do something to protect each other financially, because neither of you is immortal, and remember, we live in the real world where our relationships are not legally supported, so your slave or your owner could leave. Protect yourself financially by setting things up formally or at least informally. Enable each of you to survive and thrive should things end.

If you really like to exercise a lot of authority over the economic matters of your dynamic or you really want to hand over that paycheck and ask permission for every expenditure, you can do that. You are the ones in control of how this all works best for you. We do strongly advise that even with financial domination you think ahead about what could and will happen in the future. Make sure both of you can function on your own, and make sure you are thinking about your credit ratings and your old age. And never, ever be afraid that you are being less dominant by asking for help in financial matters.

Almost everyone needs money to survive. Our societies are built around it. Even the most independent farmer out there needs seed, animals and equipment to make her living and support her household — not to mention the time and energy she has to put into being more financially independent. The fact is that we are all interconnected in this world by money, markets, goods, and services. The two of you can't do it all by yourself. Even people living on islands interact with others, and even the hermit comes out of his cave once a year to get supplies.

What do you do when you have everything set up and you are happy with how the finances are working and life throws you for a loop? One of you loses a job. A doctor's bill isn't covered by insurance, or you don't have insurance but got into an accident. That great mortgage rate you thought you had doubles. Or things simply start breaking down around the house and need to be repaired or replaced. How do you face all that and still maintain your M/s dynamic?

The first bit of advice is going to sound familiar, and it is going to be repeated over and over in this book. Admit there are financial concerns. Be honest. Whichever of you is in charge of tracking your finances, sit down with the other or the entire household and have a blunt discussion of the facts. If you are the Mistress, you may have certain ideas about how things should be handled, but never ignore advice or suggestions from your slave. He may have had a similar experience in his past, or he may be the more fiscally prudent of you two. Making good decisions requires good information, so take your slave's input into serious consideration, and then if the situation affects your dynamic, your household or you, sure, you can make that final decision.

Whether or not you make a final financial decision for your slave will depend on how you've divided up the economics in the first place. TammyJo doesn't tell Fox he needs to go to the doctor, usually because he isn't and can't be covered by her insurance, but she has no problem pointing out when his cough has lasted too long or there's a strange mole on his back. What she can offer is to support his decisions and help him out with matters directly related to his health and personal finances.

One area she does exercise more control over is what job he has. While mostly she listens and encourages him to find a better one, she also has veto power over any job that might require that he move to another city or town. Simply put: that sort of change would radically alter how our M/s functions, and therefore he recognizes her authority, and she accepts responsibility for such an important decision. Given their difficult first year of ownership when he lived in the dorms, it would take a lot of benefits for her to approve his moving out just to take a job, and frankly the financial benefits aren't as important as our relationship to either of us.

Now our financial situation might change, and if it does, TammyJo might decide that Fox needs this opportunity in his field or that the salary and benefits are so amazing that they could just adjust to his living two hours away or only seeing each other on weekends. Right now she and he both think this is unlikely, but they know that part of making M/s work day in and day out is being flexible. Money, jobs, and spending may all require a lot of flexibility over the years. We aren't saying it wouldn't be a challenge; being flexible is challenging for many people, even in vanilla relationships. It can be harder if you set out an authority dynamic, because details about who does what, and when and how, may need to change.

Things have gotten tight, and you've made the difficult financial decisions. How do you keep the stresses of paying off that hospital bill or getting a new roof from affecting your M/s relationship? This is like a cranked-up version of the daily stresses we all can feel from just living life. Try to set aside time to just be together in ways that don't require money. It doesn't take money for him to kneel before you and give you a foot rub. It doesn't take money for her to mix up her techniques or tools in the dungeon. And it certainly takes no money for her to command and for you to obey.

Then consider ways you may have to cut into your kinky expenses depending on the seriousness of the economic situation. Why do you need a new flogger when you have five others? Use the ones you have. Why do you need to go to a convention three states away that requires flying when you have one that is two hours' drive away? Maybe it's time to look to your local community for munches instead of trekking across the state. Maybe you can go to one munch a month instead of two, or order water instead of a beer, or share an entree. If you've made friends at such events, they will still be there, and they will be understanding if you need to cut back on your kinky purchases. If you manage things well, you'll return to other venues and buy more things later. Even TammyJo, who would love it if you'd buy her books when you come to a reading or see her at a convention, understands that.

When things are good financially it can be tempting to just spend, spend, spend. Never forget that part of being in an M/s dynamic is thinking about things long-term — being committed to making this last for the foreseeable future, if you will. So even when things are great, don't make the error of just spending money like there's no tomorrow. There will be a tomorrow for you both, so always put some aside and think about what you want to do a month from now, a year from now, or a decade from now. Planning now will lessen the stress of finances later on and thus lessen the stresses to your relationship.

These financial issues are often ignored in the early stages of courtship or training, or even the early months of ownership. We think that is a huge error that many couples and households make. Sit down and compare your philosophies about money. Just as you want to be compatible in other ways, you need to determine if you can work well together financially. Are your bad money habits going to feed into each other's? Is one of you too tight with the wallet while the other always has a credit card debt? What old debts do you have? Legally or not, any financial problems or issues you have as an individual are going to affect your M/s relationship, because they affect your attitude, your health and even the time you have to spend with each other. If you have doubts early on in your courtship or training about whether or not you can make this work, don't be afraid to ask for professional advice — in this particular case a financial planner might be helpful in setting up an understanding about how your financial situation should work. Or educate yourself and try to make saving or investments a part of your life plan. The work you put in at the beginning will make things run much more smoothly in the long run.

Social Expectations

There are two types of social expectations you are going to have to deal with in your femdom relationship, and sadly they occur in both vanilla and kinky circles. The first is the issue of gender, or how you are supposed to act and think based on your biological sex. The second is how your relationship should ideally function and how it could reasonably function. In both cases our own ideas about what we should do, feel and think are heavily influenced by those who raised us and the world in which we live. Even though you might think your desires and needs are out of the mainstream, we hope you'll find it enlightening to look at just how much you still are affected by those expectations. We hope you will benefit from our advice on how to work with them or against them to enhance and maintain your M/s every day.

From the moment we are born we are raised to be either a boy or a girl, a future man or woman. Indeed, after "Are mother and child all right?" the question of whether it is a boy or girl is often the first words to roll across anyone's lips. People even have tests done ahead of time to determine the fetus's gender so they can prepare for the new arrival, and in some places people attempt to influence which sex their baby will be born, sometimes even aborting the "unwanted" one. Studies upon studies have been done trying to prove or disprove the "naturalness" of gender, and yet all one has to do is look around the world or across time to see that what is normal for one sex is quite abnormal for that same sex in another place or time. Whatever differences we may have at birth are greatly exaggerated and refined by our families and our societies. The result is that no two women and no two men are going to be the same in all their beliefs, likes, skills, or ideas.

That doesn't stop companies from trying to get us to buy things that "all men want" or that "all women crave," or to color-code toys like blocks or bears that are otherwise gender-neutral. Realizing that gender or sex stereotypes are not completely true doesn't stop you from thinking that "all men are" or that "all women are" either, if you are honest with yourself. Hopefully you didn't rush into your M/s dynamic, so you've taken the time to get to know each other as individuals, not merely a stereotype. Unfortunately, stereotypes often have a bit of truth to them, so you're liable to have to confront those expectations and ideas from time to time in your relationship.

Some of these include the idea that the man should be the primary income earner or that the man should be able to physically defend "his woman." If that is how things work out with you two, then great. But if you are trying to force each other into those roles and it is causing problems, you are dealing with gender stereotypes, not with each other at all, and you need to stop and examine what is going on.

Let's say, though, that you have dealt with these issues or you each "got over" your gender stereotypes before you got together. That doesn't mean they won't rear up with others you'll have to interact with. These can include the expectations that the man makes the decisions or that the woman will do most of the domestic work. Let's say that your friends find out that this particular man needs to "check in" before deciding to go out to the game this weekend. Charges of being "pussy whipped" are likely to be tossed about, and while that might indeed be the case in some senses — you are in a femdom relationship, after all — that accusation can hurt when it's tossed at you in public. Likewise, unthinking co-workers might whisper behind your back if they find out you hate to cook and have a man at home who does all that boring stuff.

Of course, you could keep your M/s relationship a secret, if you like; that's often called living in the closet. The problem is that secrets have a nasty way of being revealed when you least want them to be. Eventually you'll trust someone you really shouldn't or let some comment slip, or some busybody will get too nosy. So one way to deal with social expectations of how you should behave and how your relationship should work is just to be reasonably open about things and don't lie when asked about anything directly.

We aren't saying to wear your flogger on your hip when you go to the office or to flash your collar during a meeting with your supervisor — obviously neither would be appropriate. But then again, is it really appropriate to be talking about your sex life or your family life when you should be finishing a report, prepping for a class, or hurrying through lunch so you can get back on the line? The best way to deal with accusations that you aren't "normal" is to simply say "I keep my private life private," but if you do that, you then also have to not ask others for their private information.

You can also be selectively open in public settings. Because Fox is part of this family, TammyJo got into the habit of calling him her "secondary partner" (a topic we'll address more fully in the next section) when she was invited to pseudo-work events like holiday parties. It wasn't the business of her professors, colleagues, or students that she had a slave, but if it was a family invite she wasn't going to disrespect their dynamic by leaving him at home. At the more extreme end, Fox was outed at work by toxic co-workers, and he went directly to their supervisor and told her about his relationship. Doing so was damned difficult emotionally, because he feared getting fired or demoted. He is valuable enough at his job, though, that the supervisor understood and accepts that he has to check in before taking overtime or extra days at work. Such agreements aren't that uncommon among vanilla couples or families with children — work is work, but when it interferes with your family, you do have to find ways to balance it, and checking to make sure it is OK is one accepted way to do that.

For all the gender expectations and work expectations, being willing to stand up for your right to privacy or to come out a bit will go a long way toward curbing any negative consequences that may arise when folks realize you don't have the "father knows best" household. Some of you may also have the option of being in careers that are kinky themselves, or of working for yourself. But you'll still run into gender expectations.

We can't tell you the number of times that one or both of us have encountered confusion over the fact that TammyJo is the dominant in this relationship. There is still an expectation that because Fox is bigger physically he'll be the one in charge. Let's face it, some people are so concerned with their way of living that they can't see other ways of relating to others, so they attempt to force you to bend to their will through challenges or teasing or simply assuming things when they approach you. If someone treats you impolitely and it's clear that they're basing their behavior on a gender stereotype you don't fit, just smile and ignore them. Over time your calm and stable dynamic will demonstrate that there are many ways for human beings to function well, but screaming, crying, or jumping to her defense will only play into their preconceived notions of how men and women must be.

Remember when we mentioned that you've bought into some of these gender stereotypes too? Yup, you have. Take a few minutes now to fill out these sentences.

- *All men want…*
- *All women need…*
- *Girls are better at…*
- *Boys are better at…*

We bet it took you only moments to fill out those sentences. That's OK. Just because you know the stereotypes doesn't mean you have to live them. Or does it? One of the best things about being in a femdom relationship is that you have a lot of freedom to choose to follow or not follow stereotypes. Many of the things that Fox does are part of the old chivalrous model of male behavior, and some of our ways of looking at the world often do fall into stereotypical patterns, such as TammyJo needing to control the kitchen and laundry and expecting Fox to take on the outdoor chores. As long as we agree on these or they work for us with little to no frustration building up, then we can fall into these gender roles without a problem.

We can also invert them or accept that we aren't the "perfect plastic man or woman." For example, TammyJo finds it both amusing and proper that she "protects" Fox during horror movies or orders their food in restaurants. Fox loves it when she decides what they are doing and starts issuing orders. That doesn't make us less manly or womanly; it makes us who we are — and as long as we communicate and give each other positive feedback for these non-traditional gender behaviors, we feel good about them.

That raises the real issue here. Just by being in a femdom relationship, you have inverted the still-existing gender roles that men and women are supposed to have in the 21st century throughout most of the world. Details or specifics aside, boys are still raised to be in charge, and girls are still conditioned to care about others while they follow along. Sooner or later, and we hope it's later and not very often, you will find gender roles tossed into your face or into your mind, and you'll have to confront them or use them to benefit your relationship.

Relationships themselves have expectations built around them. In the next section we'll deal with the most basic of these: how many people can be in a relationship. There are other expectations as well, that have to do with religion, or that vary by region and by social class. We'll just tackle a few of the very common relationship expectations that we've encountered during our journey together. You'll see how these ideals support each other and sometimes contradict each other.

If you are in a relationship, you are supposed to be together most of the time. Actually this usually seems to happen naturally when you begin a relationship with someone new. When the passion is fresh, when you are trying to get to know each other, couples do tend to become insular and spend a lot of their time together. "Their" friends start to become "our" friends, "their" possessions become "our" possessions, etc. As long as the friends all get along and everything gets done that needs to be, then the friends are happy to include the couple and to give them space.

If you are in a relationship, you should build your life around each other. You should start to share the same religious institutions or go to shared family functions. (As a gender side note, often the woman is expected to follow the man in his career or go to more of his family events.) You should be able to describe each other as your "best friend" and buy those greeting cards that proclaim you'd be nothing without this one person. Your interests and needs are supposed to transform from his and hers into ours again... but only to a certain level, or it will be seen as unhealthy. We believe, however, that if you are in a relationship, you should still be free to be you. Being you means being able to do things at work, with friends, and with family that you've always done before. Oh, sure, others understand that your man or woman should be the center of your life, but they shouldn't be your only life. Abuse is very real; we're both survivors of abusive relationships ourselves, and we've known numerous people in abusive relationships, but there is a fine line between being in a healthy relationship where you are each other's main focus and an unhealthy one where you are the only focus. Where that line is for your dynamic depends on you both, but if you took the time to choose wisely it won't be that difficult to both build up your relationship and to stay in touch with the you that attracted your partner in the first place. Fox is a very good slave, but he's still a total science geek; TammyJo is a very powerful owner, but she still needs to just hang out with her friends. We didn't change who we are by getting into the relationship; in fact, we empowered each other to be more ourselves by having the safety and love of each other when we are together. How long will we be together? That is part of the fourth ideal about relationships.

If you are in a relationship, it should last forever. Human cultures have written poems and songs, painted and performed about the eternal love two people will share. We've also composed and performed as many songs, dramas and anything else you can name about the heartbreak of breaking up. The ideal is "until death do you part," regardless of whether or not you are married. And why wouldn't it be, if you are together all the time and building your lives around each other, but not too much? Striving toward forever is a good thing; it makes you both work, but you have to couple that with a good understanding of what a healthy relationship is for you. It may be a basic human need to be with other humans, but that doesn't mean this one human right here, right now. If forever was realistic, we wouldn't have the concepts of divorce or breakup to begin with. When things do end, as they may, we have a final and very common expectation to confront.

If your relationship ends, you should hate each other. Hate is a strong word. But depending on why and how things ended, it might apply to you. There are some exes that TammyJo hopes to never, ever see again: the mere thought makes her stomach churn. But there are others whom she continues to be friends with or at least keeps in touch with. When things end, obviously your relationship will be different, but you don't have to hate each other – or, on the other hand, to be best friends. You only have to do what is best for you, regardless of how many movies and poems tell you to do otherwise.

The biggest expectation that society has about modern relationships is the one that will assault you most directly, whether you are femdom or some other D/s or M/s orientation: Relationships should be between equals. We have all sorts of amusing or insulting names for people who get into relationships with folks who are not their equal economically or socially. We have a lot of laws built around the idea that you enter into relationships as equals and have an equal right to get out of them. Some of these laws are necessary to protect us, because abuse does happen. The truth is that relationships are not equal, because people have different backgrounds and skills. Even legally we still live in a greater society where men and women have different legal privileges and responsibilities, let alone the economic and social differences we face no matter how equal we'd like to be. As human beings we should have equal value, though bluntly that isn't how things really work yet.

But the ideal is still there in most places in the Western world. You should be in a relationship — an equal, balanced relationship. An authority dynamic innately undermines this ideal, because one of you, which means the woman if you are in a femdom situation, has the majority of the authority while the other of you, the man, recognizes her right to make decisions for you both and for him alone. So one answer to any charge that you aren't in an equal and therefore healthy or ideal relationship is to simply say "That's right," and move on from there.

You might think that this attack on the unequal nature of your relationship would come from the vanilla world, from people whose idea of BDSM comes from a movie or novel where the serial killer is described as a "master" or a "sadist." Sadly, most vanilla folks really don't care, when it comes right down to it. As long as you mind their privacy and do your job, they are more concerned with their own households than with yours. No, most attacks on 24/7 or M/s relationships come from kinky folks who aren't in these dynamics. As you've read, we argue a lot within the community of owners-slaves, owners-pets, or whatever words you want to use, but we don't generally attack each other as being in relationships that are plain, outright wrong. We've been attacked more by tops and bottoms and bedroom doms and subs at local munches and online than we are ever questioned by the vanilla people we see and talk to every day.

You could try to explain your relationship, but frankly we don't recommend it, simply because people who have so much time on their hands that they can attack others' lifestyle choices aren't interested in other ways of seeing the world. For their own reasons, they feel the need to lash out at you. You should ignore them and just live your life. Your positive, healthy M/s relationship will show itself to anyone who wants to see it. Now, if their attacks on you become public, that is a different story. Luckily, unless you are in a position of authority in some organization, you aren't likely to attract that level of attack. If you are, then again, be yourself, and if asked about your lifestyle, just state the truth.

In general that's the best way to deal with any social expectation that gets tossed into your face as an attempt to belittle your relationship, whether it's a direct, in-your-face accusation or a feeling that something isn't quite right because of something you learned in school, saw on TV, or read in the papers. All of these expectations can shake your foundation unless you take the time to establish your own personally realistic goals for your dynamic. This is why going slowly, negotiating, and even contracts are helpful. They create a new set of expectations that you can and should turn to when you don't fit the "model" of a relationship.

POLY OR MONO STRUCTURE

If you were to read some online forums or visit some munches, you might think that everyone who does BDSM has multiple partners or, alternatively, that everyone is monogamous. It's really a matter of where you are looking and who you are talking to. While we have a poly structure to our household, we don't believe it is the best choice for everyone reading this book. In fact, we think it is a very complex choice that should never be approached with any less care than you would take when getting into an M/s dynamic in the first place. We're going to try to state some of the facts as we see them about monogamy and polyamory.

The first fact is that the words most commonly used to describe one-on-one relationships versus multi-person relationships are not identical. The literal meaning of monogamy focuses on the institution of marriage — being married to one person. Beyond that it actually means being married to only one person in your entire life. Divorce and remarriage rates indicate that isn't a reality for a majority of people anymore, and historically it has also never been the reality for many people, as high death rates for mothers required fathers to remarry, and widows who outlived their husbands often wanted the economic or personal comforts of a partner.

When most people use the word monogamy now, they refer to having only one sexual partner. That isn't the reality for most of us either[1]. So within your

---

1   The Kinsey Institute, *Frequently Asked Sexuality Questions to The Kinsey Institute* (27 June 2010), <http://www.iub.edu/~kinsey/resources/FAQ.html>.

lifetime it's very likely that you won't be truly monogamous but instead serially monogamous, meaning that you'll have multiple sexual partners or spouses, just no more than one personal, intimate relationship at a time. Except that isn't quite true either, which we'll get back to shortly.

Polyamory is a modern word which means "many loves." In the Western world it cannot be related to legally recognized marriage, simply because only monogamy is legally recognized in the overwhelming majority of nations. In parts of the world where polygamy is recognized, it most often it refers to one man having several wives — an arrangement that may not work very well for a femdom dynamic. Instead what poly folks mean is that they have several intimate relationships at the same time, meaning that they might have a husband and a girlfriend, or a wife and a boyfriend, or several partners of different genders and orientations. In other words, you have multiple intimate relationships — in fact, you probably have more than you imagined.

Think of it like this.

Monogamy has three relationships at its core.

Suppose you have a monogamous relationship involving two people, A and B. This means that there are these relationships:

- *A's relationship to himself/herself*
- *B's relationship to himself/herself*
- *A and B's relationship to each other*

Total: 3 relationships.

Bet that shocked you, huh? We often forget that the most important relationship in our life is the one we have with ourselves. No matter that the social ideal is that two (or more) become one, this simply isn't the case. You don't stop being you, along with all your baggage, thoughts, and feelings, just because you have a collar around your neck or a leash in your hand. When problems arise or decisions have to be made, even in a monogamous situation, at least three different "people" should be considered — what that choice will mean for each individual, and what it means for the couple.

This principle becomes geometrically more complicated with each new person you add into a polyamorous structure. By poly here we don't mean that every person is necessarily having sex with the others or in a kinky relationship with the others, but all have connections via these intimacies that make them all function as a unit for some matters. There are many combinations possible for poly, and we'll start with a group of three just to show you how complicated things can become.

Sub-relationships in a triad:

- *A's self-relationship*
- *B's self-relationship*
- *C's self-relationship*
- *A and B's relationship*
- *A and C's relationship*
- *B and C's relationship*
- *A, B, and C's relationship*

Total = 7 relationships!

This is what we currently have in our household. Because we all live together, a good many of TammyJo's decisions are really about the seventh relationship, meaning in order to get to that she has to weigh a lot of different needs and wants. What we do together affects Tom just as what he does impacts us, and what Tom and Fox do affects TammyJo. Oh, but things used to be more complicated around here, back when we first met and TammyJo had two other submissives in training or in service to her.

We started to list all these relationships out — then we realized how much paper that would take, so we derived the appropriate formula. It turns out that the number of relationships in a given household is equal to 2^n-1, where n is the number of members. So you see, if you follow the model of a triad for a relationship with *five* individuals, you are actually dealing with $2^5-1 = 32-1 = 31$ unique relationships. 31! *Wow!* If TammyJo had stopped to think about that, she may have run screaming from the very idea of being poly at all.

Why didn't she, when she's easily accused of overthinking everything about BDSM and relationships in general? Being mono or poly, we think, is a lot like being straight, gay or bi. A huge part of it is innate desire and need. TammyJo has always been very good at thinking about and managing others. It's part of what made her a good teacher and good at leading roleplaying groups as well as maintaining leadership positions in various organizations over the years. She just seems to know how to manage, but it does require her very thoughtful work as well from time to time. It was only later, when she had to deal with some more difficult decisions, that she took the time to research group dynamics and realized what she was doing.

As the owner or the dominant in a poly situation, you do take on the bulk of responsibility in making sure things run smoothly. While it may be a very arousing idea to think of a harem of men at your beck and call, ladies, the reality is that it's a lot of work. Remember, you aren't in this alone. Each slave or submissive or even vanilla partner you have has a responsibility as well to help everything run smoothly. Furthermore, there is nothing weak about delegating authority for certain matters to one or more of the people you are in a relationship with. Give others in the poly household work to do; don't do it all yourself.

If you are the slave or submissive in a poly household, you have not only a responsibility to yourself but to everyone in that family. Jealousy is a great threat to poly, and we've seen it destroy relationships left and right, kinky or not, when it was ignored. Please try to remember that no matter your feelings, each of you entered into this relationship consensually. If you aren't poly or you find you can't handle the complications of it, then you need to excuse yourself and move on. You do not have the right to try to become a monogamous couple or reduce your quad to a triad simply because you feel insecure.

In reality, jealousy is often a fear that you aren't enough for your partner. But if you are in a poly situation, the blunt truth is: You aren't enough!

Even if you are monogamous, you aren't your partner's one and only human contact. They are going to have friends, family, coworkers, people they know from other interests, etc., and you will certainly find some of those people boring or annoying. You can never be someone's one and only; it isn't going to happen, because human beings are social creatures. This is why jealousy can plague monogamous relationships even more than poly ones.

We are in a poly structure because it works for us. We embrace the complications and struggle with them, and we've worked with and through most of the jealousies that are common in any new relationship. We want to share some basic advice about how this triad and the previous quint worked well for us.

First of all, if you are thinking about joining a poly group, be honest, brutally honest if necessary, about what you want and need. If you are dreaming of your one and only Mistress to marry and spend the rest of your life with, you have no business looking at a woman who is already with one or more people. You will end up hurting yourself if you lie to get into a poly group that you really want to break up. You might be lying to yourself first and foremost; you might think you can handle the jealousies or the time you have to share or even the fact that you have to consider someone else. Oh, you may break them up, but really, if you can break them up, do you honestly think someone else can't come along and do the same to you? You aren't that special; you really aren't. The fact is that people lie about what they want, and they are ignorant of what they need, and that is one very good reason why poly groups should go slowly when adding new people.

And that is our first piece of advice if you're already in a poly relationship: add new people slowly. This is very important. We can't tell you the number of times we've seen households ripped apart because the owner added in a new slave before the previous one was fully adjusted or the master was fully capable of handling the complexities. The reason you have to go extra slow is that you aren't adding just one new relationship, but a new person who is going to be in multiple relationships with each of the existing family members. There are going to be bumps along the way, even in the most ideal of circumstances. We strongly recommend at least three months between adding new people, and really, if you are creating a family that lives together, you may want to take a year or two between additions, since living together means that more relationships will need to be considered for any decision that is made or action that is taken.

Second, have a formal structure set up for new slaves or submissives. One way to ease everyone's stress level when new relationships are added is to get a clear sense of chores and responsibilities. This should be explicit; don't assume your new partner or your old ones just know. TammyJo always begins by pointing out that if push comes to shove, she sides with Tom, because they have a legal marriage and because they've known each other and loved each other longest. That doesn't mean that she would stay in an abusive relationship with her husband if there were one, but it does mean that the others they add to the family will not be allowed to pull them apart. Likewise, when Anna was taken on for training, she met Faith and was told that he was TammyJo's slave, and that if the three of them were together, Faith might have authority over her. Accepting training meant accepting that possibility. When Fox joined, he had two potential people who might be given authority over him. He had to weigh that before accepting the position of trainee. In general, each new person needs to know where they stand.

Some poly M/s households with multiple slaves have a formal position called "alpha," "first," or in our household, "majordomo," in cases when all the people in that household literally live together. In order for that to work well, each person needs to be clear on what their job and responsibilities are right from day one. Other households are more fluid, with the owner making that decision day to day. Finally, some function on a purely skill-related basis, where the dominant makes decisions and assigns tasks, with each slave answering only to the owner. In the past, when we've had another trainee or slave, they have functioned with Fox as majordomo, but with tasks assigned according to ability by TammyJo. We can't say how well this would work for years, because we have yet to try it beyond a few months for a variety of reasons.

Poly is easier in some senses when everyone does not live together. You don't need to think about everyone's food allergies or what their favorite TV shows are, for example, if you aren't always living the mundane parts of life together. But living apart adds other complications, such as finding time to get together or less immediate communication. Long distance relationships add another twist to things, not the least of which is an increased risk of jealousy when one partner is physically closer than another. In this era, monogamous couples may also not live together or live far away, so living arrangements and distance aren't just concerns for poly folks.

There is no one correct way to structure your household or to be poly other than this: communication needs to be ongoing and always honest. Think of how easy it is for two people to miscommunicate. That danger is only increased with each new person you add. It is very easy for the dominant or owner to become command central in terms of communication, but we caution strongly against allowing or even encouraging this. While it can feel powerful to be the central point for everyone to revolve around, it will also get tiring over time. Within our household we'd had to work on making time for Fox and Tom to talk — not joke around and discuss fun things, but actually talk —especially when one gets annoyed with the other. There are times when TammyJo just has to put a hand up and say, "Discuss it with him," then walk away.

Why would someone use their Mistress as their sounding board instead of going directly to another member of the household? Generally it is a matter of fear. We aren't talking about being afraid that the other person might hurt you, though that can happen and should be a sign that you need to re-evaluate the situation. We are talking about a fear that someone will take great offense and walk out on the household or give an impossible choice to the dominant (or to the focal person of the household, who doesn't have to be the owner, but often is in poly families). If you are generally happy in the household, if you are strongly bonded to your owner, the last thing you want to do is jeopardize everything. However, not communicating, or relying on one person to solve everyone's issues, means building resentments, and that can undermine your foundations quickly and permanently, because it destroys trust.

Poly can sound both scary and hot at the same time, and that isn't an uncommon combination of feelings to have in BDSM. Whether you go mono or poly, though, has to be a choice you each agree to, and you have to have clear expectations for either one. Never assume; always communicate. Never agree unless you are willing to put in the work and enjoy the pleasure you can have with either structure.

SEX

Ah, sex. It has so many wonderful forms and is probably one of the reasons you got involved in BDSM in the first place. It is also a potential landmine for problems in an M/s or D/s relationship, so we want to take a bit of time to discuss several problems we've dealt with over the years and heard about from other kinky folks.

One of the most common problem areas in sex is mismatched drives or desire levels. It is a stereotype that men want more sex than women. Studies show that while there are some differences between women and men in terms of how often they think about sex and the context in which they think about it, there is also a great deal of overlap between the two sexes and a great deal of variation within each sex.[2] Men are often seen as wanting sex morning, noon and night, good to go at a moment's notice. That just isn't true. There is a wide range of sexual desires, needs, and even general interest among men.

Biologically, men aren't always easily aroused or able to maintain an erection; that's why various medicines and treatments have been developed for this "problem." Is it a real problem, or simply an attempt by the pharmaceutical industry to sell more products? It is a problem if the man and his partner want to engage in particular types of sexual contact and can't, because he can't get or keep it up. If that happens in your relationship, you need to seek help, and it may not come in the form of a convenient pill, either. You may need emotional help, psychological help, or chemical help, or you may simply need to get more creative. You are in a kinky relationship after all; you should be able to be creative, right?

Women, too, vary greatly in terms of their sexual drives. In general, it does take women longer to reach orgasm than many men. Part of the joys of being a femdom and malesub is that you are in a situation where you can focus on her pleasure first, so don't worry if it takes you 20 minutes or an hour to come. Consider it more time to indulge in each other's bodies and try new things. If there are medical or emotional reasons for a woman's low sex drive, she, too, can seek professional help.

---

[2] *Frequently Asked Sexuality Questions to The Kinsey Institute.*

What neither should do is ever say flat-out "no" to any sexual contact without negotiating that with their partner. This is a common complaint in marriages — the passion just isn't there, or she/he makes excuses. Excuses are not part of upholding your authority dynamic; in fact, they threaten it with every single word. Simply saying your safeword or suddenly placing something on your hard limit list can be even more damaging if the activity or limitation seems to your partner to have come out of the blue.

Let's say that you realize that a particular sex act you've been doing with your partner actually turns you off or even causes damaging feelings or harmful physical problems. Instead of saying, "This needs to go on my hard limit list," you should ask for a time when you can talk freely and renegotiate what you are doing. This happened to us, and it wasn't handled in the best fashion, resulting in weeks and even months of negative feelings between us. You must trust your partner to understand your needs and limits, so talk to them, giving them the information they need. If your partner is the one who needs a new limit, don't push them to continue to do that sex act. If it is really important to you to do those one or two particular things, then maybe you aren't in the best match to begin with. We think you can figure out other sexual activities to do if you really care about each other and your dynamic; just make sure you talk about it before stopping any interaction cold.

One of the most common complaints we hear and read from dominant women is that there are no "real" male submissives or slaves out there; they are all just interested in sex. Second to this complaint is another one that is going to strike you as odd: he doesn't want to have intercourse as often as she does, because he thinks it is not appropriate for a slave. This is what we call a Sex Catch-22.

How did you learn about BDSM to begin with? For a lot of us, including Fox and TammyJo, we saw erotica and pornography about it and then went looking for more information. What are those genres talking about and showing? Sex! Honestly, is it surprising or even unusual, then, that men and women both see BDSM in all its forms as sexual play? No, it isn't. Not only that, but from the moment they hit puberty, and oddly even before, boys are given the message that they need to be sexual animals, and we chose that word, "animal," on purpose. Boys and men are often assumed to have blind rutting instincts that excuse and encourage sexual misbehavior. In some particularly conservative families a boy might be told he's dirty or bad for feeling aroused or doing anything about it, but more often than not his peers, male relations, and the mainstream culture reassure him that his "sin" is also perfectly normal.

To make it even more complicated, the "uniform," if there is one, for female dominants and tops is a sexy, very revealing outfit that emphasizes her breasts, ass, legs and waist. We find it particularly amusing but also frustrating when the woman complaining about how all men are only interested in sex is wearing an outfit featuring a tight corset or thigh-high boots that is focusing all eyes onto her secondary sex characteristics. Wear what empowers you as a femdom, but be realistic about the messages you are sending out.

Wearing something provocative is never an excuse for unwanted sexual attention, or frankly for anyone pretending to be interested in mowing your lawn or otherwise being of service when he really just wants between your legs. Yes, the dominant should think about the subtle and not too subtle messages her wardrobe or talk is sending, but the submissive needs to really look inside and figure out what he truly wants. There is nothing wrong with being interested in kinky sex or bedroom service, but you need to be upfront with that desire if you want to build any sort of long-term relationship.

The most common method of dealing with this "problem" of men wanting sex is the "chastity" approach. This is the idea that the woman controls the man's potential to orgasm by placing a device on him that prevents or limits erections. We have two problems with this approach for a long-term M/s relationship. The first is that it focuses on his sexuality in the first place and does so in a very negative fashion. Remember, we're talking about increasing the ability for both of you to empower your relationship to thrive for years and years. How does making a man feel negatively about his sexual feelings help him, or his dominant? By denying sex on a regular basis you run the risk of increasing its importance in the relationship by making his motivation to serve and obey centered on the opportunity to have an orgasm.

The second problem is actually health related. Some studies claim that men who ejaculate regularly have a lower risk of prostate cancer and other illnesses related to their reproductive and urinary functions, while others question these results.[3] It's hard to say which of these studies are correct, but a man who has masturbated or orgasmed regularly may find it difficult to simply quit. Of course, you may want it to be difficult, but you should do it for the right reasons, not merely because you think this is part of being in a femdom relationship. Aside from possible health issues, you can curb a man's sex drive

---

[3] S.J. Jacobsen et al, "Frequency of sexual activity and prostatic health: fact or fairy tale?" *Urology* 61(2) (February 2003): 348-53; Michael F. Leitzmann, M.D., "Ejaculation Frequency and Subsequent Risk of Prostate Cancer," *JAMA* 291 (2004): 1578-1586.

by overusing chastity. TammyJo knows a gay man whose master denied him sex for so many years that when his top wanted him to get it up, he simply wasn't able to any more. Emotionally and biologically, the years of denial had changed him. That can be a real problem when it comes to the second part of this Sex Catch-22.

What drives us both insane are the women who complain one moment about men only wanting sex and then in the next breath complain that he doesn't want to engage in intercourse. While vaginal-penile intercourse is not the best way for most women to achieve orgasm, many women still like the sensation of being penetrated. Think about how our culture has portrayed intercourse over the centuries. The penetrator, usually male, is shown as active — he is doing something — while the penetrated, usually the female, is shown as passive — she is having something done to her.

Do you remember when we mentioned that one of the problems for male submissives is this stereotype that subs and slaves are passive? If he believes that, of course he's going to have a high barrier to break though in order to perform in this fashion for his Mistress. A lot of advice is tossed about saying that one way to overcome this is to use bondage, but frankly we think that just reinforces the stereotype that men are normally the active partners in intercourse.

Instead of relying on tools to help you control or limit a man during sex, why not use your dynamic to reinforce his service and her authority? One way to do this is for the Mistress to be the one who initiates sex and makes the final decision about when and what type of sex will happen. That is probably what has been happening for the majority of your femdom relationship. Her decisions needs to be hers, not based on a self-help book, advice on the Internet, or even our book. It needs to flow from her own sexual desires.

Another way to control the sex without relying on tools or denial is to focus on the woman's body during sexual activities. Never, ever — we can't say this loudly enough — fake an orgasm, ladies. You are the one who is supposed to be in charge, so don't you dare deny your own pleasure. When you fake it, a man who isn't fully aware of how the female body works might be fooled, but even a somewhat knowledgeable man is sent the message that your orgasm isn't important. This doesn't mean you can't tease him or focus on his sexuality too from time to time, but make your satisfaction the central point of your sex life and you'll feel empowered, and you'll both be serving the dynamic, helping its authority structure grow and strengthen.

A third way to address this idea of passive and active is to realize something TammyJo's mother said that has always stuck in her mind. "If you both aren't tired when you're done, then you didn't do it right." Sex is an activity, and great sex requires a high level of activity from everyone on that bed. Activity can be in terms of physical action but also in terms of emotional connection and verbal communication. If you have difficulty thinking of new positions, then check out any number of books readily available on the topic of sex for couples. If you have trouble expressing your feelings during sex, then work on that. Make yourself be more active or less active; take charge of your sex life if you are the dominant, and learn to relax a bit more if you are the submissive.

Of course, there is the medical option to the problem. Look around you and you'll see ads for "male enhancement" and "ED" medications. While we haven't needed to rely on these sorts of aids yet, we've heard from others that they help because they increase the likelihood of erection without the stigma of blame.

Finally, one way you can address this issue of passive or dominant position is to just say, "I don't care," and enjoy it. If the Mistress is the one who wants to lie back and relax while her slave plows her, then she's exercising her authority by making those wishes known. She is ultimately the one who says, "I want this," so no one is undermining your relationship, but you are when you let the stereotype of active and passive get in your way of having a good time.

For many people, sex is not just intercourse but a full range of activities. As long as the Mistress is the one making the decisions about what type of sex to have, when and how, you are still in your femdom relationship. You haven't crossed over to the vanilla side, no matter the activity. Pornography would have us believe that a woman giving a blow job to a man or being penetrated means that she is being used. It doesn't have to be that way; in fact, it probably isn't, when you really look at who consents and who directs the activities any couple enjoys. We tried and tried to think of a particular sex act that was innately passive or active, and we were stymied, because at the foundation of any M/s dynamic is authority, and that doesn't have to change with the position or tools. If you like giving head as a Mistress, go for it; he can just wait until you are ready to let him come. If you are a slave who likes intercourse, don't worry; even if she's on the bottom tonight, her word is still your command.

Ultimately, like it or not, fair or not, the female dominant's desire for sex is what should and often does steer the course of sex in the femdom relationship. Part of the great privilege of being the one in charge is saying when, how and how often sex will happen in your relationship, or if it will happen at all. While it may be part of your authority to order some bedroom time, a good mistress will take into consideration her slave's need, desires, and limitations in the area of sex, just as she should in other aspects of their dynamic.

ILLNESS & INJURIES

Here's the reality. Both of you are going to get ill or have an injury at some point in your relationship. Unless you are amazingly lucky or have superhuman immune systems, it is going to happen. When it does happen, it can really throw a wrench into the roles you have set up, the feelings you have about each other, and your feelings about yourself.

Being healthy, both physically and to some degree mentally, is not a sign of submissive or dominant tendencies. Indeed, sometimes coping with a large number of illnesses or injuries in life makes a person more focused on being in control and on exercising control, but it can also help them see life as something they need assistance with, which can be a motivation or belief of some submissives, both male and female. Therefore, the state of your physical or mental health is not so much a sign of your kink orientation may be, but is simply one more ingredient in all that makes you you.

We want to talk about three types of health in this section and their potentially serious impacts on an M/s dynamic. We'll start with physical health, spend some time on mental health, and end with looking at how injuries and major health changes can threaten to rip your relationship apart unless you use them as another way to bond it more strongly. Please note that neither of us are qualified doctors of mental or physical health, but we do have experience with these issues. We strongly encourage you to talk to certified health care professionals about any concerns you or your partner may have in these areas. If you are afraid, we recommend the book Health Care Without Shame by Charles Moser, Ph.D., M.D. for yourself and your doctors or therapists. If your healthcare professional wants to spend more time judging your relationship as right or wrong instead of looking at the concerns you have, it's time to get a new doctor or therapist. We feel quite strongly about that.

Obviously there are at least two of you in this M/s relationship, a Mistress and a slave. You can both get physically ill, and this means that coping with that cold, flu, allergy, or even something that lands you in the hospital must take priority over your normal routine. That can threaten the dynamic you've set up if you allow it to. We're each going to talk about our own struggles with our owner-slave relationship separately, because our feelings concerning illness in each other and ourselves are different — as well as our reaction to being ill or seeing our partner sick.

TammyJo's perspective: As a dominant I have to confront this idea that I'm always right, always in charge and always self-sufficient, even though, as we've seen in this book already, none of this is realistic day-in and day-out, month after month, or year to year. I've learned to recognize my limitations in everyday life (with some minor backsliding in thought now and again). I choose to be a highly educated woman, who is a writer, who has multiple projects at any given time, and who is constantly doing something. Therefore I can choose and have chosen to delegate some matters to my slave or assign some tasks that I'm accustomed to doing personally to him to help ease the life path I have chosen. Requiring his help or service, then, is a choice in this sense as well, and it empowers me.

But I don't choose to get sick. I am notorious for not getting the rest I need or taking good care of myself, though I am learning to slow down and stop feeling like the world will collapse if I don't get something done or have to back out of an event. This is a slow learning curve for me because I see my word, my promise, as the most valuable part of my identity. Giving in to the reality of an illness can seem like a weakness, and any weakness you feel as a dominant can conjure up fears that you aren't as "domly" as you thought or that you have failed your slave or yourself. It's rather macho, actually (that's right — macho is not limited to men). Nor is it always very healthy, because pushing myself when I have a slight illness can often cause it to spiral into something far more serious. It feels like a war between my body and my mind or my desires. I have to remind myself, and be reminded, that without my body I can't do the things I choose at all. I want and need things, and thus I need to take care of my body.

A few years ago, after a long struggle with a recurring infection and a heck of a lot of testing, I learned that I had a weak immune system and have always had one, and it was probably inherited, genetic. In other words, I can take every precaution against illness, and I try to do so, but I can still get a cold, flu, or more serious respiratory illness fairly easily. This could have reassured me, made me realize that I am just a human being after all and not any sort of deity (even if my slave might teasingly call me that from time to time).

Nope. At first, it only fed those fears I still get that I'm not a good enough dominant and turned them into biological support for those fears. Interestingly, it did not suggest to me that I was submissive in any way. I mean, come on, how can you be of service to anyone if you get sick all the time? Of course, that is another stereotype I have floating around in my head and not a statement of fact, though I think you'll see some similar ideas when Fox talks about illness. Eventually, with the help of my family and friends, I came to realize that instead of a sign of weakness, this innate sickliness and my survival (indeed, my thriving for four decades in spite of it) was a sign of my strength. And strength certainly feeds into our ideas about what dominants of either sex should be.

This also proved a turning point in my attitude toward relying upon and utilizing my slave when I'm ill. If I'm strong enough to survive this constant attack on my body, then I'm strong enough to use my slave to the fullness of his potential. I have less trouble now telling Fox to do X, J, or K when I don't feel well. He's the slave; he should be making my life easier, and right now that requires that he make dinner even after a full day of work so I can sleep and get a fever down, for example. Or I'll send him to a munch to represent us all, knowing that if I go I might just infect others.

Getting to this point, and I won't pretend I don't continue to have doubts or negative feelings when I'm sick, required two types of trust we've already talked about in this book. First, a trust in myself — a solid identity as a dominant, regardless of the situation I find myself in. Secondly, a trust in my partner, in his ability to do his best, to represent me well, and to make my life easier. All those things I expect from a slave, and yet I prevented him from accomplishing them when I got stubborn and refused to take care of myself when I was sick.

My attitude toward Fox when he is sick is a bit contradictory, and as we've also said in this book, it may seem unfair at first, but M/s isn't about normal standards of fairness. First, I want him to be well. I take my job as household manager seriously and try to plan healthy meals, but I refuse to micromanage his eating to a large degree, though I have made it clear I expect him to eat breakfast and lunch on a regular basis. I also want him to exercise, and I encourage him to do so by asking if he has taken his evening walk and sometimes by walking with him. I need to be careful, though, as we discovered in the fall of 2009, because I am smaller than Fox, and the speeds he moves at are not the best for me.

Fox being healthy is a function of my affection for him as my partner and another human being, but it is also very selfish as well. If he isn't healthy, he can hardly serve me as I want or need. That leads to the contradiction about his health. I have taken care of him when he's ill, accompanied him to the doctor, and checked in to make sure he's drinking enough, but I also have an impatience when it comes to his recovery. I am no saint; I admit that — I do get annoyed when a cold makes me have to choose between his fulfilling his chores or participating fully in our nightly rituals. I think I often push him to do more than his recovery rate may suggest is healthiest, but that's one reason we still have safewords and open communication even after a decade together: I can't know what is going on in his body, so he needs to be able to tell me in some fashion. Normally, I can just see him holding his head and gritting his teeth, or the glazed look in his eyes and his pale face, and I'll see the rational decision that needs to be made. There has only been one time in our entire relationship when he ever had to safeword from an activity because of a health concern, but it will be up to him whether to share that or not with you all in the next section.

Fox's perspective: There is no shortage of experience when it comes to caring and being cared for in this household. I noted recently to Mistress that I could barely remember a year in our relationship when she has not suffered from some major injury or illness.

Shortly after I moved in, Mistress fell down the flight of stairs leading to my bedroom as she came to say goodnight. It could have been worse, but it still broke her foot and banged up her leg. There was also the illness that caused her to suffer increasingly frequent attacks of pain so severe they dropped her to her knees, the recovery from the surgery that fixed it, and the years of constant and sometimes debilitating dizziness caused by the medication needed to keep it from coming back. Most recently, there was a surgery to remove an organ that was causing her to feel as though she were starving to death no matter what she did or ate. This doesn't even cover the bad allergy seasons, the bouts of food-poisoning, or the month-long chains of flu and colds.

As Mistress mentioned earlier, she hates the feeling of dependence that being sick or injured brings (as I imagine most people do). She does everything to avoid it. Sadly, the same determination that serves her so well in most every other area of her life seems to be a marked disadvantage when it comes to her health. Mistress tends to beat back symptoms and work through the pain for as long as she can, clinging to normality and the maintenance of her self-imposed deadlines, immutable schedules, patterns of movement, etc. Sometimes she wins the day, weathering whatever was attacking her body through force of will and a handful of aspirin (and doing so without compromising any of her goals), but it used to be that she'd just hit the wall before being forced to make concessions for extended naps, reduced activity, and occasionally a visit to her doctor. Unfortunately, running full speed until one hits a wall only makes the impact worse, leading to additional frustration from the prolonged path to recovery.

What's worse, to be a slave who wants their dominant to be happy and well is to watch the process unfold — seeing the warning signs and suspecting the end result, but feeling helpless to intervene due to your role in the relationship. To me, in fact, it felt a lot like being bound and gagged — and not in the fun way. Over the years, I overcame this apprehension by looking at the situation this way: when part of your mission is to make your dominant's life as easy as possible, it is actually your duty to confront them (as respectfully and privately as possible) when they are acting in a way contrary to their own interests. I point out the warning signs, remind Mistress of the outcome, urge her to do whatever I think will avert the problem or repeat the advice we were given from the doctor the last time, and let her make the final call. Mistress still doesn't always comply, but she always listens. In those rare times when she chooses not to comply, I can still take solace in the knowledge that if the predicted problem becomes reality, I'll have a better case to make the next time.

Another thing I've noticed over the years is that when Mistress is feeling ill or is recovery from an injury, she tells everyone she comes in contact with who stands around long enough: friends, neighbors, students, co-workers, and even strangers at cons. This used to confuse me, as it seemed to go against what I already knew about her feeling like a bad dominant when in such a state, but then it occurred to me that it might be a sort of subconscious apology on her part to the people she interacted with for any shortcomings or deficiencies perceived due to not being her usual self. It also seemed to be a way of protecting herself from demands that others might make on her that could make her condition worse.

EMOTIONAL AND MENTAL HEALTH

Emotional or mental health issues are not uncommon in the general public. 26.2% of all Americans have been diagnosed with a mental illness[4] — and that's just the ones with a diagnosis. As much as we'd like to believe that we are smarter and more sane than the average American, we've seen no evidence that kinky folks don't suffer from at least the same level of mental and emotional

---

4   National Institute of Mental Health, *Mental Disorders in America* (10 May 2010) <http://www.nimh.nih.gov/health/publications/the-numbers-count-mental-disorders-in-america/index.shtml>

issues as everyone else. You are very likely to have to deal with this concern at some point during your life.

You may have to deal with it as the person with an emotional or mental health issue. It could be due to stress caused by circumstances out of your control or built up over the years. It could be something you've been struggling with for years. It could be a side effect of a physical problem or a biochemical change in your body. It could be entirely internal (acute depression, for example), partly external (the death of a loved one), or something caused by actions you've taken (such as substance abuse that has gotten out of control). You aren't alone, and we've both been there with different emotional or mental issues over the years.

This is how we've coped.

First, recognize there's a problem.

Second, be honest with your partner. Even if you don't have the words to fully describe what you're feeling, give it a try. If that Mistress or slave is worthy of sharing your life, they will try to help you and stick by you.

Third, admit you need help, and get it. You aren't superwoman or superman. If this means you see a therapist once a week, get one. If it means you need to take daily meds, take them. We may not be trained mental health professionals, but we know this: if you can't take care of your own mental health consistently, you are not qualified to be any man's owner or any woman's slave. Period.

Fourth, find a support network to help you stay on the right track. Yes, this should include your owner or slave, but it can't only be them. That's a good setup for codependency, which is not healthy. Find support groups with others who have similar problems. Keep involved in a local kink community. Attend a house of worship or social group and make friends. You don't need to tell everyone what your issues are; indeed, you probably shouldn't, but by building a network, you cultivate people whom you can turn to and who can turn to you. That sense of being supported may help you over the times when you want to blow off the next therapy session, not take your meds today, or just fall back to unhealthy behavior.

That's our short advice for what you can do if you realize you have a mental or emotional issue you need to address. We also have some advice on what to do as the partner of someone with such a concern, again based on years of experience between us.

First, don't be afraid to say that these issues may be more than you can handle. However, take some time to listen to your partner if they are brave enough to tell you they have emotional or mental issues. Do some research before you decide whether to walk away or to stay.

If you decide to stay with someone who has an emotional issue, you are going to need your own support system as well. Just as they may need therapy and a community, you are going to need support too. Remember that lots of things in life can cause mental health issues, and helping someone through theirs is certainly one possible cause. You may need different help or family/couples therapy to help you cope. If you want your own individual therapist, do not choose the same one as your partner.

Things are going to cycle from better to worse as your partner copes with their issues and works on getting mentally healthier. Even if they give it their all, there will be ups and downs. If their issues stem from years and years of problems, you are looking at years and years of work, perhaps even a lifetime. It is not easy, but it can be well worth it to be with that person as they become what they were always meant to be.

We have to end this very brief discussion of mental health issues with a sad reality. Sometimes recovering and getting healthier means learning that you aren't kinky, you aren't dominant, or you aren't submissive. That means you may have to let your partner go or transition into a vanilla relationship. We haven't had to do that, but we've known couples who have. Most D/s and M/s couples continue their authority dynamics, though, and even grow closer if they are willing to work together on one or both of their emotional issues. On the other hand, we should stress that as understanding as you may want to be, there is nothing wrong with putting limits on the amount of stress and responsibility you wish to take on with a potential partner who has a mental illness. This isn't a matter of discrimination; it's a matter of setting limits for yourself.

Aside from physical illness and mental issues, there is one final category of "illness" we need to address: injury and long-term care. Injuries happen when you least expect them. They can be a function of happenstance, accident, or your own errors. They can have a serious impact on your physical and emotional health and immediately limit you in several ways. Rarely do injuries automatically quench your D/s relationship (such as ending up in a coma). Usually, though, they are very stressful, and we'd like to address the stresses and bring up some ways we try to cope in our life together.

While working on this book, TammyJo suffered an injury as well as a strange illness that resulted in her having her gallbladder removed. Both required serious adjustment in how she lived her daily life and provided us both with a test of how our relationship could continue to function.

Beyond the feelings of being weak or requiring help that a dominant or submissive commonly feel during general illnesses, long-term health issues provide even more challenges. Psychologically, they can be draining. While you can always tell yourself that you will get over the flu or your medication can help with the allergy season, an injury or a long-term illness means that your life changes for months, if not longer. Normal divisions of chores and duties, normal eating habits, and even the amount of income you might be able to bring in may change. We want to share just a few of these issues that we have personally dealt with.

TammyJo injured her hip when she over-exercised in the early fall of 2009. After changing all of our diets and putting herself on a great exercise program, she doubled her workout without proper build-up. She has this tendency, and even though Fox and Tom both tried to remind her to be careful, like many dominants she ignored his advice to her detriment. The resulting pain, lack of exercise, and even serious slowing down of her basic ability to walk produced massive feelings of stupidity, inadequacy, and fears that she'd gain back all the weight she'd lost and be robbed of all the improvements she'd made in her general health. These feelings killed off her sex drive and made her grumpy and demanding, running Fox ragged and fueling his general feelings of inadequacy as well.

A similar situation arose in the winter of 2010 just as she had worked her way back up to about 90% of her exercise regime. This time she was almost crippled by serious and constant abdominal pain, which turned out to have been caused by gallstones. It took months of testing to find that out, though, because of trying to match her busy schedule with doctors' busy schedules, and finally she needed surgery, which didn't go as smoothly as we had hoped. Unlike with her previous injury, she literally felt out-of-control because no one could say why this happened, other than it seems to run in her family and gallbladder problems are fairly common in the USA. Feeling out-of-control, feeling like there is little you can do, will kill a dominant's desire to command or even accept service, let alone exercise her sex drive or energy to play with bondage or SM.

For Fox specifically and submissives in general, it's not much better. Fox felt absolutely helpless. He and her husband tried everything they could think of for weeks, but there was nothing that either could do to even ease the pain for very long. Fox's feelings of helplessness and frustration with himself gradually made it harder for him to even be around her. When TammyJo was finally able to get tested and act on her doctor's instructions, these things she could actively do gave her a small feeling of control. After the surgery, she needed Fox and

Tom's assistance with even the most mundane of tasks, such as showering, putting laundry into the machine, and retrieving items from low shelves, as well as higher ones. Being able to help again was all it took to make Fox feel a great sense of relief, but for TammyJo, his service was tainted in her mind by the realization that she needed the help.

That is the biggest struggle that all types of illness present to any dominant. Commanding someone because you want to feels empowering; getting their aid because you need it feels annoying at best. Being served can be hot until it is no longer a choice you make but assistance you require. You are not alone when you feel this way, but honestly, even knowing that may not help much.

We wish we had the answer to how you can deal with these issues of illness and injury, short-term and long-term care, but the truth is that we struggle with this ourselves, and we did even as we were writing this book. Here are some basic suggestions from our own struggle.

Mistresses who are ill or injured need to admit it to themselves and to their slaves. Try to come up with a plan for what to do when you are sick or injured. If you can, decide what chores you will turn over to your slave and think of ways he might offer help without seeming to take charge of the situation. Just telling him that you'll need your medicine (and when), help with dressing, or even reminders not to do any heavy lifting, for example, can be put into the context of new instructions for him to follow. Be very wary of doing too much too soon, because you might end up sicker or more injured than before. You think it's hard to have to rely on your slave for two weeks? Imagine what it will be like if you end up harming yourself so badly that it takes months to recover.

Slaves who are ill or injured have a tougher psychological hurdle to overcome in several ways. It can be hard to tell your owner what you need, so why not take her to the doctor with you so she can hear the directions, warnings, and suggestions herself? Try to be honest about what you can and can't do. It is very tempting to say, "I'm not that sick," and go about your daily tasks, then end up feeling much worse with your Mistress standing over you with a frown, demanding to know why you didn't tell her that you were running a fever or had a headache or pulled a muscle. Telling her is risky, because she may not care, but the odds are that, if you both want this to be a long-term M/s dynamic or perhaps a lifetime relationship, she cares a great deal about your physical and mental health and will consider what is best for you. If on the other hand you have an owner who doesn't seem to care about your well-being at all, we suggest you might want to reevaluate that relationship.

Illnesses and injuries that result in lifetime changes can be incorporated into your D/s by focusing on what is important for your dynamic. If your dynamic's core is that the owner has the final decision, she can still do that, but may have to limit it to certain areas or simply construe her decisions as going along with what is needed because she is wise enough to see that it must happen this way. If providing mundane service is your core, then find different ways to do the same services, or find other chores you can do. For example, being in an accident where you end up in a wheelchair will indeed affect your ability to drive or garden, but maybe you can take over other tasks or arrange to hire help without your owner's direct guidance. If your relationship flows around any particular type of interaction, you may have to find other ways to express your dynamic. Better still, be varied in how you express the authority in your relationship and how you offer submission, so you can always find ways to keep things going, even under difficult conditions.

Family & Friends

There are two general categories of family and friends you are likely to deal with while in your femdom relationship. First, those whom you grew up with and see in your mundane lives. Second, other kinky folks whom you choose to associate with. We want to talk about how being in a femdom relationship can be both challenged by and reinforced by both types of connection.

The family you were born or adopted into has expectations for you, voiced or not. We bet that those expectations did not include either owning another human being or being owned by someone. TammyJo is out of the closet, and yet her original family doesn't know much about her relationship with Fox. How can she be out of the closet then? The name you see here on the book is the name you'd find her scholarly works under and the name the IRS knows her by. It is her name; she isn't hiding, but she also knows that different people need and want different information. Her parents never told her much about their intimate lives, and as long as they don't ask she doesn't give them the details, beyond the fact that Fox is part of her family. Fox's parents know about as much, but he isn't out; Fox isn't a name you'd find on any legal records about him. He chooses to be more private for his own reasons, but he is out to some degree just by being with TammyJo.

If your family, parents, sisters, brothers, or other relatives ask questions about your relationship and they don't seem to know much about BDSM, we recommend you tell them in vanilla terms that you are together and part of each other's lives. If you have gotten married, odds are they won't ask much beyond knowing that. Most people we know who have come out to a relative or two have had fairly neutral experiences. We've heard of some terrible reactions, and Fox's sister's reaction wasn't particularly good. Over the years, as long as you demonstrate your positive relationship, you may find, as Fox has, that even those relations who were afraid or worried for you start to accept it as your valid choice.

We've also heard of some very positive reactions — people whose parents turned out also to be kinky, or they discovered that an uncle was into that, too. Or their family simply helped support their dynamic by inviting their partner to family gatherings and treating them like they did everyone else. We used some gendered terms there on purpose, because so far the most positive examples of coming out to family have come from male-dominant couples or same-sex couples. Given the social expectations that still exist for men and women, it might be that femdom is a bit too odd, or maybe all of you are still hiding in that closet, so we haven't heard many good stories yet.

Family wants two things from you. First, they want you to be healthy and happy (usually; let's not get into abusive families in this book, as that would take an entire tome to tackle in relation to BDSM or alternative sexualities). If your family's only information about kink has been the mainstream media, they have good reason to be worried when you come out to them. Let's face it — we aren't shown in a positive light most of the time, and the best we can often hope for is comedy, rather than a serial killer who calls himself a "master." We found a great book that may have helped Fox's sister come to accept our relationship and which we've given to friends who've had concerns as well.[5]

Handing someone a book, however, is not going to do everything. You have to be willing to be open with someone with your information, as well as loyal to your relationship when you talk about it. Trust us, there are times when the questions are going to get so rude or seem so repetitive that you might want to scream at your family, but maintain your cool. Reacting in such an intense fashion will only feed their worries. Ultimately and sadly, if they refuse to listen and are not interested in your well-being and happiness, you may have to choose between your Mistress or slave and them. Their inability to adjust to your reality reflects the second expectation your family has for you.

---

5   Dossie Easton and Catherine A. Liszt, *When Someone You Love Is Kinky* (Emeryville: Greenery Press, 2000).

As much as they want you to be happy and healthy, though, they also have familiar expectations for you that can range from time you spend with them to following in the family business. They've had a picture in their minds from the time you were born of their little baby girl or boy growing up to do or be something. This can be something simple, such as "a good woman with a good husband," or complex, like "a doctor with three kids." When you don't match that ideal they've created over the years, it will obviously hurt them. Just like wanting you to be happy and healthy, they may perceive this expectation as wanting what is best for you. Be yourself; show them that where you are now in this femdom relationship is what you want. Don't just use words; use your actions — include your slave in family events, or include your Mistress in discussions with your family. You don't need to be on high protocol; in fact, you probably want to fall back on how you'd act at work or with vanilla friends. You can be in your M/s relationship and still be with your family.

Friends are very similar to relatives in many ways, though it will depend on how close you were to each friend or the type of friendship you have. Anyone who comes to our home is "warned" that we live in a non-traditional family, and if they have a problem with that, they probably shouldn't come over. Over the years very few potential friends have fled from us. In fact, just by being out and being ourselves around our friends, we've learned that a fair number of them are also kinky or have thought about some kinky activities. None of them live 24/7 like us, and few of our close friends routinely engage in kink, but they know we are safe people to talk to if they have questions. Even people TammyJo went to high school with aren't shocked, because really she's the same person, just more confident and more grown-up.

Friends can be family you choose, so remember that: You choose them. This means you don't have to tolerate them if they attack your life or your partner. Reach out to your friends who are struggling with your decision to be in an M/s dynamic just as you would your family, but try to make some other, more understanding friends as well.

Some cities have several kinky groups. This was the case when TammyJo and Tom lived in NYC. Yet most people don't have the time or money to attend everything. They find themselves in the same couple of groups, making friends with regulars. The result is very similar to living in a small community with only one or two kink organizations. The friendships' common interest is their kink, sometimes with the same orientation, sometimes across orientation. We've been friends with other poly families, with maledom couples, with gay men, and with all sorts of people through the years. It is nice to have someone you can talk to about all the stuff that even your coolest vanilla friends may not really grasp.

These kinky friends can be reassuring when the vanilla world is dragging you down. They can be a great resource to learn new techniques or to generate new ideas from. They offer the normal socializing benefits of a vanilla club with the benefits of being more open about what happens behind your closed doors. However, these friendships are not immune to the problems any groups, couples, or organizations can have.

Just like your family and friends, your kinky buddies are interested in your health and happiness, but they also have expectations for how your life should be. Some may go so far as to tell you that doing things your way is the wrong way. Others may attempt to "rescue" your partner from you. Generally this "one true way" mentality will show itself in a few weeks or a few meetings, we hope well before you've formed any deep emotional bonds. If someone is offensive to you or yours, you need to walk away. Having kinky friends can be great, but it isn't necessary to a stable, long-term femdom relationship. Lots of us live with very few kinky friends in our lives, and we live just fine. Our biggest support comes from the liberal-minded vanilla friends we interact with each week, because they know we are merely expressing our affection for each other in a different way.

Family and friends, however, can see things that those in the relationship can't. While we are big supporters of the idea that everyone who wants to be in a 24/7 situation has the right to be in one, we also know that abuse can hide under the guise of kink. If several of your family members or friends, kinky or mundane, are coming to you with the same or similar concerns, you may want to think about what they are saying. It can be very easy to not recognize the emotional and psychological abuse that makes excuses for bruises or insults. But if your personality changes for the worse, your friends and family may be the ones in the best position to notice that. Whether you are on the top or the bottom, take to heart what your friends and family say if they come to you with a serious concern. You don't have to follow their advice, but a strong, healthy D/s dynamic will not be destroyed simply because you took some time to reflect on what is going well and not so well.

Then there are work friends, or colleagues, as we prefer to think of them. With so many of us working full-time, it can be easy to see your fellows in the office or the trenches as your friends. Indeed, they may be your friends outside of work hours. But the amount of personal information you provide or ask about may be different from what you give an old school buddy or your sister. As cycles of economic boom and bust should show us, work is work, and even those great friends can disappear if you lose your job or there is competition for a position. In general, we don't recommend being more out than necessary at work. Fox had to come out to deal with some rumors at his job and to set up the protocols for his working overtime. TammyJo often had to do pseudo-casual things like dinners and parties with her department when she was in university that were supposed to include the entire family. None of these people needed to know that she owned Fox or that he had to answer to her because he is her slave. All they need to know was that we have family obligations and that we expect the same consideration they'd give anyone else.

Of course, you might work in a kink-related job, like in a store, on the production line for sex toys, as an artist or writer (like TammyJo), or as a web designer (like Fox). Those work friends are people you may want to be a bit more open with about your relationship, because knowing you are also different from the mainstream may land you the job to begin with or help you work your way up in it. Business is still business, though, so we suggest not having the same expectations for those you work with as you do for your other friends and family. Your boss may think you are a great bondage model and love to hear your stories, but the fact remains that she'll lay you off when the clients just aren't lining up. Keeping your expectations realistic in the work environment will help you cope with all manner of changes there.

The fact is that most vanilla people aren't that interested in what we do as long as we are good daughters, sons, business partners, friends, or whatever. The same is true for most kinky folks. Be an honorable person, have confidence in your relationship, and show the world the positives, and you'll find yourself supported far more than attacked. Your loyalty needs to be to your dynamic first and foremost if you want it to thrive for a long, long time. So if people are attacking you or your partner unjustly, you need to distance yourself from those people.

Examples of Everyday D/s and Ownership

To use us as an example, here is what our average day looks like from the aspect of maintaining our authority dynamic.

TammyJo gets up the earliest, usually, and goes about getting her breakfast, reading the paper and doing anything online she needs to do. If she sees that

Fox is up, she'll call down to him, "Good morning, boy!" and he'll reply, "Good morning, Mistress!"

Before he leaves for work, Fox checks in to kiss her and wish her a good day, adding Mistress, not her name. She reminds him of any plans they have or any errands she may want him to do after work. If she has an errand for him in the morning, such as dropping off something at the post office, Fox makes sure to build that time into his waking up, breakfast, and driving schedule.

The bulk of the day they are out of touch, because TammyJo is busy on several projects, and Fox isn't supposed to have his phone on at work. They think about each other on and off, perhaps making plans for the evening or a weekend.

If Fox is asked to stay longer at work or come in on a day he was not scheduled for, he will call TammyJo during his break and ask if he can take on that extra time — generally by inquiring if she had plans for him those times. He may also call to ask if he can have time to run by for a haircut or to go shopping on the way home. They abide by her decision, which is made considering everyone in the household.

When Fox gets home, he greets her and inquires about her day while she does the same; their language is the only thing that really separates this from vanilla life in any large fashion. If she requires or wants his help with dinner or any chores, she will tell him then. He either obeys immediately or requests some downtime to recover from his day (again abiding by her decision on the matter) and tries to smile while he works, even if he wishes her decision had been otherwise. The odds are that he'll be groped or spanked at some point during this preparation, simply because he's there and she can.

We all eat as a household, talking about our days and bitching about politicians or stupid people on the news. TammyJo asks everyone for a report on their day, and we all listen to each other, offering feedback that we hope is supportive.

If there are chores after dinner, those are assigned, but normally Fox has a few hours of privacy to unwind while TammyJo spends time with Tom or other friends. Often we schedule time to watch a TV show or a movie together most evenings, with Fox fetching anything we want or even cuddling up together. Occasionally he sits on the floor at her feet while they watch.

Fox is often dismissed again until it is TammyJo's bedtime, since she is not the night owl he is. They take that time to discuss anything of importance or interest; they have a nightly ritual they go through where they center on their dynamic and reaffirm their commitment to it. They part knowing that they are fulfilled and empowered by her authority and his obedience.

That might have been so boring for many of you to read. Where were the whips and chains? Where was the begging and screaming? Where were the hot orgasms?

Those happen — just not every day. We have play time and sex, and we make special plans to do complex scenes. That's wonderful, but those times are not what fuels this relationship day in and day out.

Instead we are strengthened by continual use of some rules, rituals, and protocols and our open acceptance of each other's needs and desires. We affirm each other's position through our language and our concern daily and in small ways. Those are the things that will give you the power to last a lifetime.

8

PARADOXES OF OWNER-SLAVE DYNAMICS

Using and Needing Your Slave: The Paradox of Ownership

Fox and TammyJo once hosted a discussion of people who lived M/s relationships as part of their everyday lives at a regional leather convention a few years back. More than thirty people attended. Out of those people, only one said he purposely designed his relationship with his slave so that he never used him for anything he really needed, because he felt a master shouldn't need a slave. The use of the word "need" or "depend" can make some people on the dominant side of things very uncomfortable, because it clashes with their concept of what being an owner is.

Too often we rush into M/s or D/s relationships with our minds full of porn or erotica, following our groins over our heads. Let's get one thing straight: A Mistress needs a slave. Period. You can call yourself an owner, a Mistress, a Master, or High Lady of the Great Heavens if you like, but that's just a title.

The position, the role of being the owner in a lifetime M/s dynamic, requires that you have someone to exercise your authority over. You can debate and decry the use of the idea that you need your slave, but the cold hard fact is that you do. The degree of need you have will depend on the dynamic and what you expect from each other.

Beyond just needing him so you can exercise that authority that turns you on and fulfills some inner drive you have as a dominant, you may also grow to need your slave emotionally. Some dominants work hard at not developing particular emotions for their slaves, especially anything they might call love. We've noticed over the years that you can control your actions, and to some degree reprogram your reactions, but it's very hard to stop or control your emotions. If you start feeling affection you don't think is proper for a Mistress to have about her slave, we challenge you to stop and really reflect on where you got this idea. Is holding that idea that you must distance yourself, that you can't need your slave, actually limiting your ability to make the commitment necessary to help an M/s dynamic thrive and survive for years? Remember, there are many types of love, and some type is necessary, or you simply will not put the effort required into this lifestyle.

Financially needing a slave often seems less of a paradox if you believe the online ads and come-on lines. There are plenty of ads out there for financial slaves, both on the female and male side of things. Finances are a need you'll have whether you are a couple or not. In some M/s dynamics, it's more of a vanilla het marriage sort of setup where the owner makes the money and controls it, while the slave stays at home. In others the income the slave makes is part of his service to his Mistress. In most relationships these days, you all have to work and contribute something financially, and that doesn't change just because he's wearing your collar.

The biggest challenge, the real underlying challenge to the idea that you, the Mistress, need your slave, is that it feels as if it makes you less. Does it? There is a difference between needing someone you choose to be with and being dependent on someone for your very existence. There are times when Fox is a great help to TammyJo and she wonders what she might do without him. Ultimately she knows she could do all those things herself. That she allows him to do those things, that she uses him for those things, feels like a sign of being strong now, because it's admitting she's just a human being with limitations and a good selfish streak as well. She knows herself well enough to know that consensually owning a slave is part of what she needs to feel fully herself.

TammyJo says, "Knowing myself well enough to go against almost everything the greater society around me tells me I should want has got to be some of the greatest strength I've ever known. I'm lucky that I found Fox and that he has submitted to me so fully." And yet, Fox embodies the other paradox we want to close our book exploring.

ACTIVE SUBMISSION: THE PARADOX OF SLAVERY

What does it mean to be a slave in this world where men and women are almost equals? What does it mean to be a slave in a world where the idea of slavery seems so horrible on every level? It means you have to want it, you have to need it, and in short, you have to actively pursue it.

As we discussed before, a lot of people think that being a slave means just waiting around for orders and just doing what you are told, or that being submissive is being passive or unmanly. Submission in an M/s relationship that is going to last a long time is more a bending of your will to the other person and to the relationship itself. It is an action you choose to take and which, if you are in a healthy relationship, will start to feel natural and normal to you. Every single time a man kneels at a woman's feet he is doing something the greater society deems silly at best and abnormal at worst. Conscious or not, it is a choice he makes every day.

It is also a choice the Mistress makes every day as well, and in order for her to make that choice she has to feel that it's worth her time and energy, that it's fulfilling to be the owner. Slaves help by being active in their submission: figuring out what turns her on, what you can do to make her life easier, and how to give her positive feedback without necessarily taking a time-out to say, "You're doing great." That is active submission.

You can call it whatever you like. Just see it as a more submissive state or just being yourself, but as the slave you are half of what makes this all work. You are vital to the next year, the next decade, the entire lifetime as an M/s couple or household. If you hold yourself back, if you only react instead of acting, you might be holding back your relationship, not allowing it to go deeper into you as a person.

Ultimately being a slave isn't a collar around your neck or a contract. It's feeling so connected to that other person that you put them over yourself without consciously doing so, and in that you actively begin to serve and feel truly fulfilled. It may happen with several people or with only a few. For all our talk about how there isn't "the one," you may actually have one relationship in your lifetime where you fully feel both a man and a slave. When you feel that balance, you will know what active submission is.

Your concept of M/s is really the key here. Your relationship needs to be structured around what you think is appropriate for an owner and slave. We hope our book has shed some light on how one couple, one household, has merged their ideas of M/s so that they both feel fulfilled and expect to continue to be fulfilled for the foreseeable future in this authority dynamic. If it works for you, both of you, then it works, and we don't want you to change a thing. If you're struggling, then we think our experience might open your mind so you can re-examine what you both want and work on making his kneeling at her feet one of the best relationships of your life.

TAMMYJO'S CONCISE ADVICE FOR FEMDOMS

Learn to be selfish, not uncaring.

Wear what makes you feel confident and dominant.

Never agree to more than you can handle.

Get a lot of experience — seek out training and mentors.

Practice new techniques.

Laugh at your mistakes.

Embrace saying "I'm sorry."

Note your successes and celebrate them.

Be honest about your limitations.

Accept service in all its forms.

Acknowledge his good work, and correct problems fairly.

Do not be afraid to ask for help.

Accept that you can't change him fundamentally.

FOX'S CONCISE ADVICE FOR MALESUBS

You have limits, even if you don't realize what they are yet.

Get a lot of experience — seek out training and mentors.

If it looks or sounds too good to be true, it's probably fiction.

Dominants are not telepathic — make issues known before they become problems.

Relationships require constant effort and communication — D/s ones doubly so.

Allow yourself to stretch a little. If it isn't beyond your limits, go along with it.

Try to learn a broad range of services, from erotic to domestic.

Keep in mind that your actions and behavior in public reflect on Her.

Try not to let your mistakes crush your self-esteem. Learn from them and be better.

Note your successes and celebrate them.

Do not be afraid to ask for help.

Enjoy the ride.

APPENDIX: SAMPLE CONTRACTS

Sample Contract[1]

#1 **Names/Titles:**

The slave may not, at any time in scene (private or public), call Owner by Her name or any first name that She is known by. Owner will be called "Mistress" at all times; in public he is to use discretion, and when referring to Her to Her colleagues, family, and friends who do not know of this contract, Her given name "TammyJo" may be used.

The Owner may call the slave anything she wishes at all times; in public She is to use discretion, and when referring to him to his colleagues, family, and friends who do not know of this contract, either his community name "Fox" or his legal name is to be used. slave's formal scene name = Sterling.

#2 **Schedule:**

Living Under Separate Roofs: Time is to be made to see each other on a regular basis depending on work and school obligations. Both Owner and slave acknowledge that they need personal time as well for friends, themselves, family, and other relationships. However, this contract signifies the importance of this relationship and thus they will make time for face-to-face time as well as a consistent line of communication via phone or email. Owner will not demand more time from slave that She feels he can safely give Her and he will communicate his needs and schedule to Her in advance so that this can be achieved.

Living Under Same Roof: Since both Owner and slave will see each other on a daily basis, the following responsibilities and expectations will apply. slave has the right to his own space and time to himself to pursue his own leisure, academic, personal, and relationship matters, though he will keep Owner aware of these activities in general terms so there are no scheduling conflicts. slave will show Owner the proper respect at all times when seeing Her in their home, offering his services and expressing his desires when he is not engaged in other activities listed above. slave will trust his Owner's judgment to do what is best for him in regards to the amount of time his services take and the amount of time he needs for his personal and professional life.

---

[1] Used by TammyJo and Fox for both training and their first three years as owner and slave. It still forms the basis of any training TammyJo is inspired to do.

#3 Mutual Obligations: Both slave and Owner know that the other (or alters as the case may be) may have other scene relationships or romantic relationships. Out of respect for this relationship (which is consider to be "primary" for the slave and "secondary" for the Owner) they will inform each other of the pursuit of such relationships, taking into consideration the feelings and concerns of each other and making sure such other scene/romantic relationships do not interfere with their own commitment.

#4 Privacy: Both Owner and slave will respect each other's privacy by not "outing" the other to family, friends, or colleagues who do not know about this contract. Likewise they will not attempt to read or view any personal materials unless given permission.

#5 Owner's Obligations: Owner agrees to administer fair discipline, respect limits, honor safewords, insure safety, provide for slave's basic care while fulfilling her right to have Her desires fulfilled under the boundaries of consensuality.

#6 slave's Obligations: slave agrees to be quick to obey any command but to ask questions if uncertain of how to perform a task; to always perform to the best of his ability, use titles when appropriate, to practice attentiveness, to honor Owner's safewords, to offer care and comfort, to communicate to the best of his abilities, and to show Her proper respect in all ways while reserving the right to protect himself, his academic career, his family and his friends. slave will use his safewords will thoughtfulness and sincerity, preferring honest communication to express his needs, desires, and concerns.

#7 Honesty: Both Owner and slave must be completely honest in all dealings with each other. Tact, however, is a beneficial route.

#8 Duration of Contract: This document will be the formalized basic of ownership from the day it is signed through one (1) full year. At that, if another contract is desired it will be renegotiated.

#9 Ending this Contract: Ending of this contract will occur if 1) unnegotiable differences arise, 2) breaking of hard limits or disrespect for safewords occurs, 3) drastic changes in lifestyle of one party which necessities renegotiation.

"I understand and agree to uphold this document to the best of my ability."

Owner: _____ Date: _____

slave: _____ Date: _____

Sample Training Contract[2]:
Program of General Training for Bottoms and Submissives

This program combines practice and experience to help some determine limits, appropriate roles, and how to adapt to different styles and degrees of BDSM interactions.

General Training:

I. Self-Improvement:

a. Readings in both fiction and non-fiction from the Trainer's library and the public library will be assigned.

b. Trainee is to purchase a journal of some type to write in. These writings are to be done immediately after a session is completed (Trainer will provide ten minutes for this in her home), the day after a session, and at any point the Trainee wishes to comment upon what they feel, think, or read in relationship to BDSM.

1) The Trainer may ask for an entry to be read to her or merely shown to her to demonstrate that the journal if being kept. However, the Trainer will respect that this is a private matter for the Trainee's own growth and not make comments upon it beyond training purposes – Trainee is to say whatever is in his/her mind.

II. Instruction in general areas of "Service":

a. Furniture: offer body to serve as chair, table, footstool or other inanimate object; may also be used as a punishment and when used as such, no verbal responses, other than safewords, are allowed

b. Worship: a gentle kiss or series of kisses on an object or body part for as long a time as dictated by Trainer

c. Butlery: offering food, drink or other objects for Trainer's use; each item should be presented in a manner which maximizes the Trainee's physical attractiveness and minimizes the Trainer's work; may also include cooking for the Trainer and her kink-friendly spouse since cooking and housework may be required in a number of D/s relationships

d. Dressing/Undressing: caring for clothing of the Trainer and of her

1) passive = simply hold Trainer's clothing for her or fold them after she disrobes and place them where appropriate

2) active = physically aid Trainer in her dressing or undressing; coats should always be helped on and off then hung up in the appropriate place

---

2   Used by TammyJo for many, many years.

e. Grooming: includes bathing, hair care, and nail care; bathing requires preparation of tub and water as well as actual attendance during bath and aid with washing and drying

f. Sexual: Trainee should be prepared to give any type of sexual service, within both parties' limits, and to offer himself to Trainer at all times, but he/she should never expect that Trainer will use him/her thus; indeed no direct sexual involvement (actual touching of one partner's sexual organs by the other) will be allowed by this contract prior to 45 days of completed training (such contact will be discussed at this point and detailed out in writing)

g. Massage: a skill needed for every trainee; all means (practice, reading, classes, video watching) necessary to learn and maintain this skill at a high level must be undertaken by the Trainee under guidance of the Trainer though any expenses incurred will be the Trainee's responsibility; this service may also be offered in public as a way to show affection or to introduce subtle public scening but confirmation of both parties is required

h. Manual Labor: household chores or carrying bags or packages; can be a valuable part of subtle public scening because it looks so vanilla

i. Secretarial: taking notes, reading passages out loud, answering of phone, or editing of Trainer's work, taking all care to be respectful in any criticisms

j. Entertainment: composed from various elements that may be either ordered or offered for Trainer's amusement:

    1) story telling — either alone or playing off of each other's words in an interactive verbal scene

    2) singing — should be done only if Trainee's voice is pleasing

    3) comedic performances — should be in good taste, which is, of course, dependent upon Trainer's and Trainee's opinions

    4) juggling or other physical feats

    5) games — while playing, Trainee should attempt to make sure Trainer wins or that she is offered compensation should she lose

    6) dancing — either for or with Trainer, in public or private; when in private it should be done in a manner meant to attract the Trainer and present the Trainee in as beautiful and available way as possible

III. Experiences in forms of SM or Sensory play:

Trainer and Trainee will experiment in a wide range of SM activities including but not necessarily limited to the following: flogging, spanking, bondage, caning, hot wax, ice, enemas, shaving, tickling, CBT, sensory deprivation, knife play, etc.

a. Purpose is twofold:

1) to introduce the novice Trainee to the range of BDSM experiences in a safe environment so they can better understand what they like and what their limits are

2) to introduce both Trainer and Trainee to each other's limits and interests in an interactive and enjoyable manner.

Specific Training:

I. Trainee Positions: (these may be adjusted for physical handicaps)

Position #1: Kneeling on both knees, head to ground, just touching Trainer feet/shoes, palms flat on ground by head.

a. to be used to greet Trainer at beginning of scene

b. to signal that Trainee wishes to begin a scene

Position #2: Kneeling on both knees, back and neck straight but eyes not looking directly into Mistress', thighs spread, palms resting flat on thighs. Alternative form: standing with legs spread shoulder width apart, hands clasped behind lower back, head slightly bowed.

a. at ease position

b. to receive collar

Position #3: Standing up straight, hands clasped behind neck, eyes forward, legs spread so that feet are shoulder width apart.

a. inspection position

Position #4: Same as #2 but palms flat and together and offered toward Trainer.

a. to offer any object for her use or inspection

Position #5: Same as #2 but hands crossed at wrists and offered, palms upward, to Trainer.

a. to inform Trainer of any disobedience for which Trainee knows he/she should be punished

b. to express the understanding that a punishment has been earned and is accepted

Position #6: Kneeling on both knees, thighs spread wide and pelvis tilted forward, arms crossed behind back so that chest is thrust forward, head tilted up to expose neck

a. to offer body to Trainer for use as she sees fit

b. to express own physical desires

Position #7: Kneeling on both knees, hands on floor, ass tilted up, thighs spread wide, back arched

a. to offer body to Trainer for use as she sees fit

b. to express own physical desires

Position #8: At Ease: stand in a designated place with arms resting behind back, feet at a comfortable distance apart, watching the Trainer in a relaxed but attentive fashion. Speaking when spoken to is permitted, as is offering services if the need arises.

Other positions are simply responses to services being rendered or those taken at owner's instruction. Trainee should always aim at presenting himself/herself in an attractive and respectful manner.

These formal positions may not be changed or deviated from until

1) physically moved by Trainer

2) tap of Mistress' right foot means to move to next position in numerical sequence

3) tap of Mistress' left foot means to change back to previous position

4) verbal command to assume another position, called either by number or a basic description of its function/use

5) necessity toobey other commands or to offer service

II. Interviews: The Trainee is expected to conduct a series of short interviews with the Trainer in an attempt to learn her needs and desires. Notes should be taken and kept for the Trainee's continued information. Such interviews may be conducted in person, over email, or over telephone, in scene or out of scene.

a) interviewing of potential play partners is always a great idea so these can be considered practice for negotiation in the future

OTHER BOOKS FROM GREENERY PRESS

BDSM/KINK

... But I Know What You Want: 25 Sex Tales for the Different
James Williams $13.95

The Compleat Spanker
Lady Green $12.95

Conquer Me: girl-to-girl wisdom about fulfilling your submissive desires
Kacie Cunningham $13.95

Erotic Slavehood: A Miss Abernathy Omnibus
Christina Abernathy $15.95

Family Jewels: A Guide to Male Genital Play and Torment
Hardy Haberman $12.95

Flogging
Joseph Bean $12.95

The Human Pony: A Guide for Owners, Trainers and Admirers
Rebecca Wilcox $27.95

Intimate Invasions: The Ins and Outs of Erotic Enema Play
M.R. Strict $13.95

Jay Wiseman's Erotic Bondage Handbook
Jay Wiseman $16.95

The Kinky Girl's Guide to Dating
Luna Grey $16.95

The Mistress Manual: A Good Girl's Guide to Female Dominance
Mistress Lorelei $16.95

The New Bottoming Book
The New Topping Book
Dossie Easton & Janet W. Hardy $14.95 ea.

The (New and Improved) Loving Dominant
John and Libby Warren $16.95

Play Piercing
Deborah Addington $13.95

Radical Ecstasy: SM Journeys to Transcendence
Dossie Easton & Janet W. Hardy $16.95

The Seductive Art of Japanese Bondage
Midori, photographs by Craig Morey $27.95

The Sexually Dominant Woman: A Workbook for Nervous Beginners
Lady Green $11.95

SM 101: A Realistic Introduction
Jay Wiseman

21st Century Kinkycrafts
edited by Janet Hardy $19.95

GENERAL SEXUALITY

A Hand In the Bush: The Fine Art of Vaginal Fisting
Deborah Addington $13.95

Love In Abundance: A Counselor's Advice on Open Relationships
Kathy Labriola $15.95

Phone Sex: Oral Skills and Aural Thrills
Miranda Austin $15.95

Sex Disasters... And How to Survive Them
C. Moser, Ph.D., M.D. & Janet W. Hardy $16.95

Tricks... To Please a Man
Tricks... To Please a Woman
both by Jay Wiseman $13.95 ea.

When Someone You Love Is Kinky
Dossie Easton & Catherine A. Liszt $15.95

TOYBAG GUIDES:
A Workshop In A Book $9.95 each

Age Play, by Bridgett "Lee" Harrington

Basic Rope Bondage, by Jay Wiseman

Bondage Rigging, by Nickels *(coming Spring 2011)*

Canes and Caning, by Janet W. Hardy

Clips and Clamps, by Jack Rinella

Dungeon Emergencies & Supplies, by Jay Wiseman

Erotic Knifeplay, by Miranda Austin & Sam Atwood

Foot and Shoe Worship, by Midori

High-Tech Toys, by John Warren

Hot Wax and Temperature Play, by Spectrum

Medical Play, by Tempest

Playing With Taboo, by Mollena Williams

Greenery Press books are available from your favorite on-line or brick-and-mortar bookstore or erotic boutique, or direct from The Stockroom, www.stockroom.com, 1-800-755-TOYS.